A Practical Guide to
Office Gynecologic
Procedures

A Practical Guide to
Office Gynecologic
Procedures

Editors

Paul D. Blumenthal, MD, MPH

Professor
Director, The Stanford Gynecology Service
Department of Obstetrics and Gynecology
Stanford University School of Medicine
Stanford, California

Jonathan S. Berek, MD, MMS

Laurie Kraus Lacob Professor
Chair, Department of Obstetrics and Gynecology
Stanford University School of Medicine
Director, Stanford Women's Cancer Center
Stanford Cancer Institute
Stanford, California

Contributing Editor

Mary T. Jacobson, MD

Clinical Associate Professor
Department of Obstetrics and Gynecology
Stanford University School of Medicine
Stanford, California

. Wolters Kluwer | Lippincott Williams & Wilkins
Health
Philadelphia · Baltimore · New York · London
Buenos Aires · Hong Kong · Sydney · Tokyo

Acquisitions Editor: Rebecca S Gaertner
Product Manager(s): Nicole Walz, Amy Dinkel, Ashley Fischer
Production Project Manager: Priscilla Crater
Senior Manufacturing Manager: Benjamin Rivera
Marketing Manager: Kimberly Schonberger
Designer: Doug Smock
Illustrator(s): Jennifer Smith, Sara Krause
Compositor: Aptara, Inc.
Printer: C&C

© 2013 by LIPPINCOTT WILLIAMS & WILKINS
Two Commerce Square
2001 Market Street
Philadelphia, PA 19103 USA
LWW.com

Printed in China

Library of Congress Cataloging-in-Publication Data

A practical guide to office gynecologic procedures/[edited by]
Paul D. Blumenthal, Jonathan S. Berek.
   p. ; cm.
  Includes bibliographical references and index.
  ISBN 978-1-60547-704-6
  I. Blumenthal, Paul D. II. Berek, Jonathan S.
  [DNLM: 1. Diagnostic Techniques, Obstetrical and Gynecological. 2. Ambulatory Care–methods. 3. Genital Diseases, Female–diagnosis. 4. Genital Diseases, Female–therapy. 5. Gynecologic Surgical Procedures. WP 141]

  618.1'075–dc23

2012049415

To our patients, for offering us the privilege of caring for them and the opportunity to improve the techniques described here and especially for their patience as they shared the time it takes to teach the next generation of healthcare providers.

To Dr Antonio Scommegna and the attending staff at the late Michael Reese Hospital and Medical Center for providing a cauldron of clinical experience and the inspiration for lifelong learning and teaching.

To the late Dr. Irv Cushner, Professor of Obstetrics and Gynecology at UCLA for both his enduring wisdom and his support of women's health.

To the late Dr. Kenneth J. Ryan, the Kate Macy Ladd Professor of Obstetrics and Gynecology, Harvard Medical School, the Brigham and Women's Hospital, for his guidance and adherence to ethical principles and equality in the arena of women's health.

Contents

1 PAIN RELIEF FOR OFFICE GYNECOLOGIC SURGERY   1

Thuong-Thuong Nguyen and Paul D. Blumenthal

2 EXTERNAL GENITALIA   6

3 VULVAR INTRA-EPITHELIAL NEOPLASIA   15

Katherine Fuh and Paul D. Blumenthal

4 BARTHOLIN'S GLAND CYST/ABSCESS   17

Anahita Jafari, Mary Jacobson, and Paul D. Blumenthal

5 CONDYLOMATA AND MOLLUSCUM CONTAGIOSUM   23

Anahita Jafari and Paul D. Blumenthal

6 EXTERNAL GENITALIA: TOLUIDINE BLUE TESTING IN VICTIMS OF SEXUAL ASSAULT/ABUSE   30

Katharine Anne Willoughby and Harise Stein

14 ENDOMETRIAL BIOPSY   92

15 ENDOMETRIAL IMAGING   99

16 ABORTION   114

17 INTRAUTERINE INSEMINATION   131

18 TRIGGER-POINT INJECTIONS: ABDOMEN, BUTTOCKS, AND SKIN   135

19 HYSTEROSCOPIC STERILIZATION (ESSURE)   140

Contributors

Paul D. Blumenthal, MD, MPH
Division of Family Planning Services
and Research
Department of Obstetrics and Gynecology
Stanford University

Laura Brodzinsky, MD
Division of General Gynecology
Department of Obstetrics and
Gynecology
Stanford University

Pauline Chang Yu, MD
Department of Obstetrics and Gynecology
Stanford University

Carrie Frederick, MD
Division of Family Planning Services
and Research
Department of Obstetrics and Gynecology
Stanford University

Brooke E. Friedman, MD
Division of Reproductive Endocrinology
and Infertility
Department of Obstetrics and Gynecology
Stanford University

Katherine Fuh, MD
Division of Gynecologic Oncology
Department of Obstetrics and
Gynecology
Stanford University

Stephanie Gustin, MD
Department of Obstetrics and
Gynecology
Stanford University

Paula J.A. Hillard, MD
Section on Pediatric and Adolescent
Gynecology
Department of Obstetrics and
Gynecology
Stanford University

Mary T. Jacobson, MD
Division of General Gynecology
Department of Obstetrics and
Gynecology
Stanford University

Anahita Jafari, MD
Department of Obstetrics and
Gynecology
Stanford University

Jessica Kassis, MD
Department of Obstetrics and
Gynecology
Stanford University

Inna Landres, MD
Department of Obstetrics and
Gynecology
Stanford University

Kevin Henry Maas
Department of Obstetrics and
Gynecology
Stanford University

Leah Millheiser, MD
Division of General Gynecology
Department of Obstetrics and
Gynecology
Stanford University

Thuong-Thuong Nguyen, MD
Department of Obstetrics and
   Gynecology
Stanford University

Christine C. Picco, MD
Department of Obstetrics and Gynecology
Stanford University

Eric R. Sokol, MD
Division of Urogynecology and Pelvic
   Reconstructive Surgery
Department of Obstetrics & Gynecology
Stanford University

Harise Stein, MD
Division of General Gynecology
Department of Obstetrics and Gynecology
Stanford University

Irene Wapnir, MD
Chief of Breast Surgery
Department of Surgery
Stanford University

Katherine Anne Willoughby
Department of Obstetrics and
   Gynecology
Stanford University

Amy E. Wong
Department of Obstetrics and
   Gynecology
Stanford University

Foreword

As gynecologists, we frequently perform office procedures because the medical conditions that we see on a daily basis demand proper and prompt diagnosis, evaluation and treatment. Most of these procedures have the benefit of simultaneously accomplishing these aspects of patient management. The essential aspects of care are that they be done correctly with the least discomfort to our patients and only when necessary. Conducting these procedures in an office setting can save time and money, while improving the outcome for our patients.

This book describes and discusses the most commonly used office gynecologic procedures. The goal is to facilitate optimal management of our patients and their gynecologic problems. Written by the faculty, fellows, and residents of the Stanford Department of Obstetrics and Gynecology who took great care to include the details for the performance of excellent office-based diagnosis and treatment, this book is an important tool for practitioners of our specialty.

I extend my gratitude to Dr. Paul Blumenthal and my colleagues for this valuable effort and their commitment to outstanding patient care.

Jonathan S. Berek, MD, MMS
Laurie Krause Lacob Professor and Chair
Department of Obstetrics & Gynecology
Stanford University School of Medicine
Director, Stanford Women's Cancer Center
Stanford Cancer Institute
Stanford, California

Preface

LOGISTICS OF OFFICE-BASED PROCEDURES

The obstetrician—gynecologist performs a variety of diagnostic and therapeutic procedures in daily practice. While, traditionally, the operating room has been the preferred venue for many procedures, an increasing number are carried out in the ambulatory setting. Indeed, in the past 10 years, the number of office-based procedures in surgical fields has doubled from 5 to 10 million cases. The principle advantage of the office setting is the ability for the physician to provide care in an expedited fashion in an environment controlled by the clinician, at a time and location that is more convenient for both the provider and patient. In turn, this may allow for more rapid diagnosis and treatment. Not only is the time needed to schedule an operating room saved, but performing a procedure in the operating room with the numerous admission, setup, and discharge requirements is considerably more time consuming than when performed in the office. In addition, particularly in today's environment of increasing healthcare costs, physicians are aware that it is commonly more cost effective to perform a procedure in the office and the reimbursement for office-based procedures may be greater than that for hospital-based procedures, potentially making them more profitable for the practitioner. Finally, the patient may find it more comfortable to undergo procedures in the office and provide the patient with a better healthcare experience.

As office-based procedures become more widespread and are relatively free of the regulation-constraining hospital procedures, physicians must be adequately trained in order to assure procedures are performed safely and expeditiously. This begins with proper patient and case selection in order to minimize procedural risks. In the event of a complication, the physician and the office should be prepared with emergency equipment, medications, and resources such as swift and easy access to a hospital. This is especially true in procedures that require moderate sedation, necessitate close patient monitoring, or that have the potential for hemorrhage. Professional judgment and experience is required to make the decision, when needed, to abort the procedure for reasons such as inadequate pain control, excessive bleeding, and other unanticipated complications.

The purpose of this manual is to serve as an informative, "need-to-know" clinic reference for gynecologists, family practitioners, advanced practice clinicians, and residents. The indications and technique of commonly performed office procedures are reviewed, along with practical information such as patient positioning, anesthesia and equipment needed, and aftercare. In addition, the relevant Physician's Current Procedural Terminology (CPT) and International Classification of Diseases (ICD-9) codes are listed.

The procedures reviewed in this guide can all be safely and effectively performed in the office or clinic setting by a proficient practitioner. For all procedures, including those not listed in this guide, proper informed consent must be obtained. Although it may be tempting to minimize the risks of a procedure performed in the office, it is important to remember that they may actually be greater than if the procedure were performed in the hospital. However, with the proper preparation and resources, office-based procedures can be safely and efficiently performed and be a more cost-effective and patient-friendly mode of providing healthcare. This guide aims to assist the practitioner in achieving this goal.

Amy E. Wong, MD
Paul D. Blumenthal, MD, MPH

Acknowledgments

It has become fashionable to say that it "takes a village" to achieve anything, and in this case, that village was principally populated by two women who took seriously the part of their job description that says "other duties as requested." Without their persistence, cajoling, and attention to detail, this book would not have been possible. We are therefore very grateful to Kelsey Lynd and Alma Gonzalez for their efforts in helping create this work and their commitment to women's health.

We gratefully acknowledge the staff at Wolters Kluwer Health Lippincott Williams and Wilkins, particularly Ashley Fischer who willed this book into existence, Sonya Seigafuse who recognized its possibilities, and Nicole Walz who shepherded it through a long adolescence.

Finally, we want to thank our residents and fellows at Stanford, a truly outstanding group of young physicians, who are obligated to learn at least one new thing every day. While preparing the material contained in this guide they went beyond the call of duty and thus, learned to be teachers, too.

Pain Relief for Office Gynecologic Surgery

Thuong-Thuong Nguyen and Paul D. Blumenthal

OVERVIEW

When performing procedures in the office, pain relief in the form of analgesia, local anesthesia, and moderate sedation is often necessary. In the sections that follow general approaches to these methods are provided. General principles associated with the use of local anesthetics and moderate sedation are discussed. Since they have specific uses related to specific procedures, pudendal and paracervical blocks are discussed elsewhere (see Chapter 10, Pudendal Block and Chapter 13.7, Cervix: Paracervical Block).

RELEVANT ANATOMY

- Dependent on specific procedure performed.

PATIENT POSITION

- Dependent on specific procedure performed.

LANDMARKS

- Dependent on specific procedure performed.

ANESTHESIA

Preemptive analgesia: Analgesia administered prior to the procedure to prevent or reduce intra- and postoperative pain.

- Ibuprofen 600 to 800 mg po
- Ketorolac 30 to 60 mg IV
- Gabapentin 600 mg po
- Clonidine 4 mcg/kg po

Local Anesthesia

- Lidocaine 1% (10 mg/cc), maximum of 3 to 5 mg/kg without epinephrine or 7 mg/kg with epinephrine

- Epinephrine at 1:100,000 can decrease blood loss and systemic dissemination of lidocaine via vasoconstrictive effect of epinephrine
  - Adding 1 cc of 8.4% sodium bicarbonate buffer to every 10 cc of lidocaine can decrease pain associated with injection of the normally acidic lidocaine
  - Side effects: Transient numbness or tingling of lips and tinnitus
  - Toxicity: Arrhythmias, seizures
  - Onset of action within 5 minutes, duration 0.5 to 2 hours
- Bupivacaine 0.25% to 0.5%, maximum 1 to 2 mg/kg without epinephrine or 3 mg/kg with epinephrine
  - Advantage: Longer duration: 2 to 4 hours
  - Caution: Higher concentration more painful upon injection
  - Side effects and toxicity: Arrhythmias and cardiac arrest
  - Avoid in hypoxic or acidotic pregnant women
- Mepivacaine 0.5% to 1%, maximum of 4 mg/kg or 280 mg
  - Advantage: Longer duration: 1.5 to 3 hours
  - Disadvantage: Poor fetal hepatic metabolism, therefore avoid in pregnancy

EQUIPMENT

- 24- to 30-gauge needle
- 5- to 10-cc syringe
- Alcohol swabs

TECHNIQUE

Subcutaneous or intrafascial injection of local anesthetic prior to skin incision or puncture:

1. Insert the needle, bevel up, at a 25- to 45-degree angle into the skin.
2. Once in the subdermal tissue, aspirate to ensure that the needle is not in a blood vessel to avoid intravascular injection of anesthetic.
3. If no blood returns on aspiration, slowly inject anesthetic to create a wheal beneath the dermis.
4. Once the dermis or subcutaneous component is anesthetized, deeper tissues can be injected if the procedure requires it.
5. Allow 2 to 5 minutes for onset of anesthesia.
6. Please see Chapters on Pudendal and Paracervical nerve blocks.

MODERATE SEDATION

Moderate sedation: A combination of analgesia and anxiolysis that decreases consciousness. The patient maintains ability to breathe spontaneously, communicate, and follow commands.

- Common uses: Termination of pregnancy (dilatation and curettage, dilatation and evacuation, manual vacuum aspiration), cervical cone biopsy, incision and drainage, biopsy, fulguration, hysteroscopy, laparoscopy, in vitro fertilization
- Contraindications: Physical abnormalities which could compromise airway access, American Society of Anesthesiologists status 3 to 5, respiratory infection, prior sedation complications or failure

- Risks: Over sedation, respiratory depression, aspiration, seizures, arrhythmias, phlebitis
- Requirements: Knowledge of correct medication doses, how to manage complications, and basic life support, especially airway management and oxygen administration. (Note: Many hospitals and outpatient surgery centers require the clinician to pass a written or online module in moderate sedation as part of privileges accreditation.)
- Patient evaluation:
  - Complete history and physical examination, and if indicated by health status or procedure: ASA status, CXR, EKG.
  - A light snack on the morning of the procedure and small sips of clear liquids alone or with pills 2 or more hours prior is acceptable. If NPO status was recommended to the patient prior to the procedure but oral intake is documented, this is not necessarily a contraindication to providing moderate sedation.
  - Risk and benefits reviewed. Procedural consent signed.
  - Escort available for postprocedure care and transportation.

RELEVANT ANATOMY

- IV access either by direct injection, heparin lock or intravenous line.

PATIENT POSITION

- Dependent on specific procedure performed.

LANDMARKS

- Dependent on specific procedure performed.

ANESTHESIA

- See equipment list for complete list of medications.

EQUIPMENT

- At least two personnel
  - The operator responsible for the provision of the conscious/moderate sedation
  - A licensed RN, PA, NP, MD, DO, or DMD to monitor the patient's vital signs, pain scale, and sedation scale during the procedure
    - Vital sign monitors: Continuous pulse oximeter, blood pressure cuff
    - Oxygen per nasal cannula or face mask
    - Advanced airway support equipment available in office/clinic
    - Cardiac defibrillator available in office/clinic
- Sedatives
  - Diazepam (Valium) 0.5 to 2 mg IV bolus. Can start at lower dose and slowly titrate up by 0.5 to 1 mg every 2 minutes
  - Midazolam (Versed) 2.5 to 5 mg IV bolus. Can give 2.5 mg every 2 to 3 minutes.
    - Advantage: Faster onset, results in retrograde amnesia
- Narcotics/opiates
  - Morphine 1 to 2 mg IV boluses up to 5 to 15 mg
    - Onset of action 5 to 10 minutes, duration of action 3 to 4 hours
    - Advantage: Longer duration

- Side effects: Bradycardia, hypotension, precipitates bronchospasms in asthmatics
- Fentanyl 50 mcg IV, followed by additional 25 mcg in 2 to 3 minutes if needed
  - Onset of action in 1 to 2 minutes, duration of action 30 to 60 minutes
  - Advantage: Faster onset, less nausea
- Remifentanil (Ultiva): Initial 1 mcg/kg over 30 to 60 seconds.
  - Onset of action in <1 minute, duration 5 to 10 minutes.
  - Advantage: Faster onset
- Meperidine
  - Less commonly used due to side effects and drug interactions
- Antiemetics
  - Metoclopramide 10 mg IV
  - Ondansetron 4 mg IV
  - Ranitidine 50 mg IV or other H_2 blocker IV can be given preoperatively
- Medication reversal
  - Naloxone (Narcan) 0.4 mg, for opiate-induced respiratory depression
    - May need additional dose for meperidine due to longer half-life
    - Must observe patient for 1 hour after administration
- Flumazenil (Romazicon) 0.2 to 5 mg in increments of 0.2 mg every 1 minute for benzodiazepine-induced oversedation
  - Must observe patient for 2 hours after administration

TECHNIQUE

1. Document an "anesthesia plan" including assessment and grading of airway, examination of heart and lungs, and ASA risk category.
2. Achieve IV access and have monitoring devices (pulse oximetry and BP monitor) ready.
3. Administer the opioid, sedative, and antiemetic.
4. Monitor and record the patient's vitals and level of sedation and pain carefully.

REQUIREMENTS FOR DISCHARGE HOME

1. The patient should be alert and oriented.
2. Vital signs are within normal or acceptable limits.
3. The patient has been monitored for the appropriate time if a reversal agent was administered.
4. Pain levels should be less that 4 out of 10 with 10 being the worst imaginable pain.
5. There is a responsible adult who will escort the patient home and watch for complications.
6. The patient is given written instructions regarding postprocedure care, when to seek medical attention, and a phone number to call in case of emergency.

AFTERCARE

- Postprocedure pain control
- NSAIDS:
  - Acetaminophen 650 to 1,000 mg po q6h prn
  - Ibuprofen 600 mg q6h prn or 800 mg q8h prn

- Narcotics:
  - Hydrocodone-acetaminophen (Vicodin) 5/500 1 to 2 tabs po q4—6h prn
  - Oxycodone-acetaminophen (Percocet) 5/325 1 to 2 tabs po q4—6h prn

PEARLS

- "Verbacaine"/"Vocal Local": A verbal/conversational stream of dialogue that distracts the patient from pain during the procedure has been shown to decrease the patient's level of perceived pain.
- Ethyl chloride can be applied to the skin to anesthetize it prior to injection of local or introduction of intravenous line.
- Experience indicates that, when possible, allowing or even encouraging the patient to watch her procedure while it is ongoing (e.g., during office hysteroscopy) provides a level of distraction that also results in reduced perception of pain and lower required levels of sedation.

Punch Biopsies for Vulvar Lesions

Stephanie Gustin, Laura Brodzinsky, and
Paul D. Blumenthal

Vulvar biopsy is a simple office-based procedure that allows for prompt tissue diagnosis and subsequent directed management. Lesions that warrant biopsy include the following:

- Lesions that are enlarging or changing in color or appearance
- Dermatoses unresponsive to treatment leading to doubt regarding diagnosis
- Raised or pigmented lesions
- Lesions with associated white or thickened areas
- Any lesion that is suspicious for malignancy

RELEVANT ANATOMY

The vulva is a collection of external mucocutaneous structures comprising the female genitalia. Located between the thighs, the vulva is bounded anteriorly by the mons pubis, posteriorly by the posterior commissure, laterally by the labiocrural fold, and medially by the hymenal ring (Fig. 2.1.1).

PATIENT POSITION

- Lithotomy

LANDMARKS

- Important anatomic landmarks include the mons pubis, labia majora, labia minora, clitoris, urethral meatus, vestibular glands, Bartholin's glands, vaginal vestibule, and hymen.
- Landmarks are principally important for documenting the site of the biopsy and the suspected pathology, based on location.

ANESTHESIA

- In almost all cases, simple injections of local anesthesia in the form of 1% lidocaine (or similar) and/or the use of ethyl chloride in the area immediately surrounding the lesion in question will suffice for provision of pain relief.

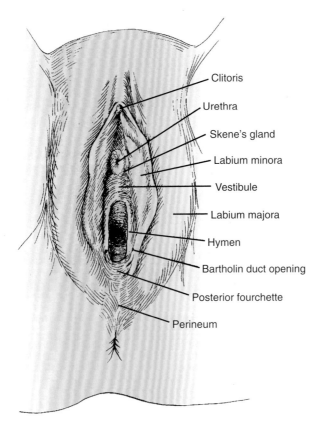

FIGURE 2.1.1 ● Vulvar anatomy. Vulva and perineum—view of external female genital anatomy showing the various structures. LifeART image copyright © 2012 Lippincott Williams & Wilkins. All rights reserved.

EQUIPMENT (Fig. 2.1.2)

- A punch biopsy kit such as a set of Keyes dermal punch biopsy rings
- 1% lidocaine (3 mL is sufficient) and ethyl chloride spray
- 5-mL syringe and a 22-gauge needle
- Topical disinfectant, such as Betadine, alcohol, or iodophor
- Silver nitrate or Monsel's solution
- 4.0 Polyglactin (e.g., Vicryl or similar) suture
- Adson (or similar) tissue forceps
- Dissecting or iris scissors

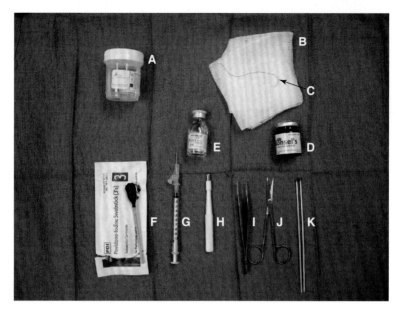

FIGURE 2.1.2 ● Sample instrument tray for vulvar biopsy. **A:** Small formalin container for specimen, **B:** Gauze sponges (4 × 4), **C:** Cutting (skin) needle with suture, **D:** Monsel's solution for hemostasis, **E:** 1% lidocaine, **F:** Topical disinfectant, such as Betadine or alcohol, **G:** Syringe with high gauge needle for local anesthetic, **H:** Keyes punch biopsy instrument, **I:** Fine tissue forceps, **J:** Dissecting or iris scissors, **K:** Silver nitrate sticks.

TECHNIQUE

1. Upon identification of a site requiring biopsy, cleanse the skin using alcohol, Betadine, iodophor, or other appropriate disinfectant.
2. Inject a small amount of local anesthetic (usually 1 to 2 mL of 1% or 2% lidocaine is sufficient) under the lesion, achieving a wheal in the immediate area. Make certain to aspirate prior to injection of local anesthetic. Alternatively, ethyl chloride can be sprayed onto the area from whence the biopsy will be taken. This can reduce the discomfort associated with the injection of lidocaine and sometimes is sufficient anesthesia for very small biopsies (Fig. 2.1.3).
3. Upon confirmation of anesthesia, direct the Keyes punch biopsy perpendicular to the skin, such that you are entering the skin straight on.
4. Begin rotating the biopsy clockwise and then counter-clockwise, this will assist tissue penetration (Fig. 2.1.4A).
5. Once the blade portion of the tool is no longer visible, remove the Keyes biopsy instrument by pulling outward, away from the skin.
6. A small circular hole with a core of tissue will be visible. This tissue sample penetrates below the dermis into the subcutaneous tissue.
7. Carefully grasp the tissue core with Adson (or similar) forceps.
8. Gently retract the tissue to reveal the base of the tissue, which is usually still connected to the subcutaneous tissue.
9. Free the connection by cutting across the base using dissecting scissors (Fig. 2.1.4B, Fig. 2.1.4C).

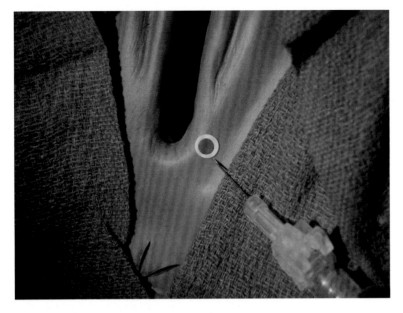

FIGURE 2.1.3 ● Injecting local anesthetic under area for biopsy.

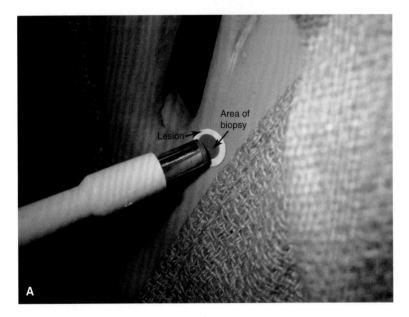

FIGURE 2.1.4 ● Biopsy of vulvar lesion with Keyes punch. Instrument is rotated in place to incise tissue. **A:** Biopsy instrument being placed over specimen to be excised (red dot) from the total lesion (yellow dot) under which anesthetic has been injected. *(continued)*

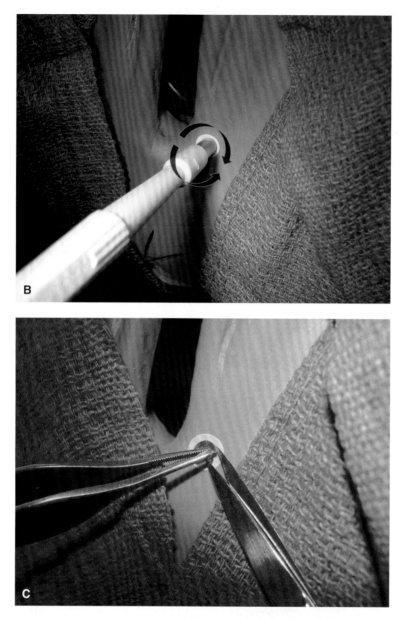

FIGURE 2.1.4 *(Continued)* ● **B:** Biopsy instrument in place over area to be excised. Using rotation (*arrows*) and pressure, the skin will be incised and the biopsy specimen created. **C:** Adson forceps used to lift specimen (red dot) away from skin as it is cut away from lesion (yellow dot) using iris scissors.

10. A small amount of bleeding may be evident upon excision of the tissue core. A combination of direct pressure, and/or use of Monsel's or silver nitrate are generally sufficient to create hemostasis.

11. If the aforementioned treatments do not provide hemostasis, placement of a single interrupted suture may be necessary.

AFTERCARE

- Instruct the patient to keep the area clean using gentle soap and water.
- Administration of triple antibiotic cream and/or ointment may be used to prevent infection.
- Acetaminophen or ibuprofen should be sufficient for pain relief.

CPT Codes
56605.   Biopsy of vulva or perineum (separate procedure); one lesion
56606.   Biopsy of vulva or perineum (separate procedure); each separate additional lesion (list separately in addition to code for primary procedure)

PEARLS

- Biopsy is often not performed soon enough in the process of workup and treatment. Given the ease with which it can be performed, it should be used early on in the diagnostic or confirmatory process.
- Persistent or intractable bleeding may indicate a cancerous growth. Admission for packing and observation is rarely necessary.
- Biopsy of the clitoris or the urethra in the office is not recommended unless adequate pain relief can be assured (clitoris) or management or potential urologic complications (urethral fistula) can be managed.

Q-tip Test for Vulvar Vestibulitis

Stephanie Gustin, Laura Brodzinsky, and
Paul D. Blumenthal

Vulvodynia is a diagnosis of exclusion, as it is a pain syndrome without an identifiable cause. It is important to differentiate generalized as opposed to localized vulvodynia, as this can lead to a more prompt and accurate treatment strategy. Cotton swab testing can be used to map the vulva and establish the pain pattern.

RELEVANT ANATOMY (Fig. 2.2.1)

PATIENT POSITION

- Lithotomy

LANDMARKS

- The vestibule is the innermost area of the vulva. It is immediately external to the hymenal ring, extending along the labia minora from the clitoris down to the most inferior aspect of the vaginal introitus (Fig. 2.2.1).
- The vestibular glands, from whence vestibulitis may emanate are contained throughout the vestibular area, contained just under the mucosa.

ANESTHESIA

- No anesthesia required.

EQUIPMENT

- Cotton swab

TECHNIQUE

1. With the patient in the lithotomy position, begin by first gently swabbing at the 2 o'clock position of the vestibule. When pain is present, ask the patient to rate the pain as mild, moderate, or severe (Fig. 2.2.2).

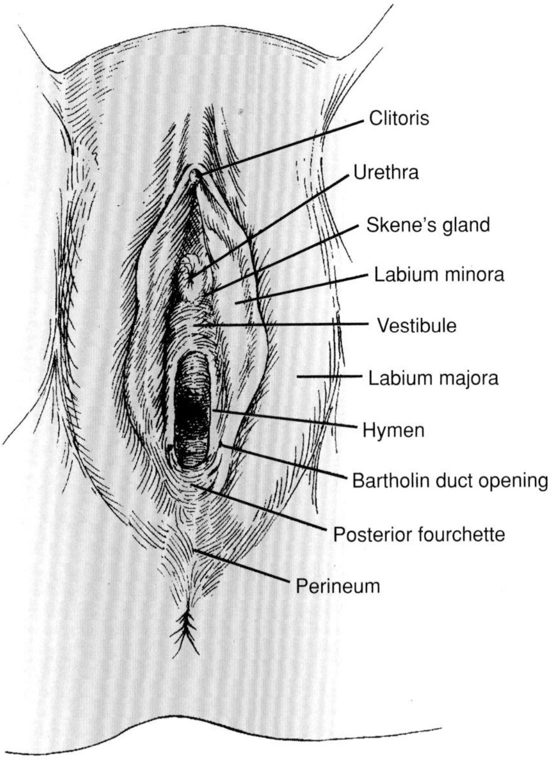
Clitoris
Urethra
Skene's gland
Labium minora
Vestibule
Labium majora
Hymen
Bartholin duct opening
Posterior fourchette
Perineum

FIGURE 2.2.1 ● View of external female genital anatomy showing the vulva and perineum. LifeART image copyright © 2012 Lippincott Williams & Wilkins. All rights reserved.

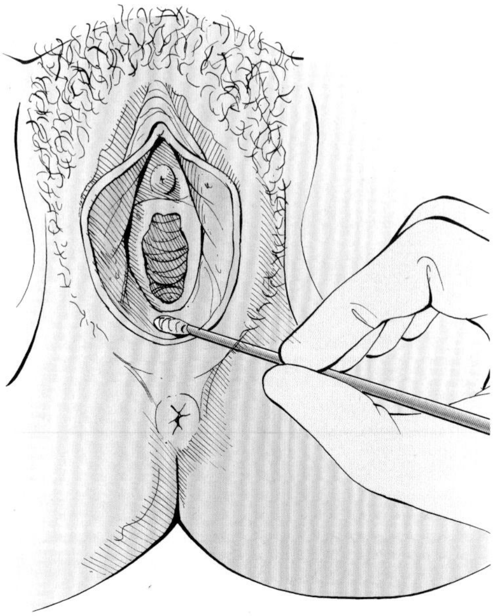

FIGURE 2.2.2 ● Q-tip being use to probe for vulvar sensitivity. From Haefner HK. Critique of new gynecologic surgical procedures: surgery for vulvar vestibulitis. *Clin Obstet Gynecol* 2000;43(3):689–700.

2. Proceed to the 4, 6, 8, and 10 o'clock positions, qualifying the pain at each region.
3. Document your findings on a map, which can be used to evaluate disease progression or regression over time.

AFTERCARE

- None

CPT Code n/a

PEARLS

- Testing the vestibular area for trigger points should be undertaken gently and slowly enough to allow the patient to differentiate one tested area from another.

Vulvar Intra-epithelial Neoplasia

Katherine Fuh and Paul D. Blumenthal

Vulvar intra-epithelial neoplasia (VIN) was reclassified in 2004 replacing the previous VIN 1, 2, 3 format. "This disorder is now classified into two main groups: VIN, usual type, which contains: the former subcategories (1, 2, 3), VIN warty type, VIN basaloid type, and VIN mixed (warty, basaloid) type; and a second group classified as VIN differentiated type which comprises the former category simplex type. VIN differentiated type accounts for 5% of VIN, typically occurs in postmenopausal women, not associated with HPV and more associated with lichen sclerosus. VIN usual type is more commonly associated with HPV."

RELEVANT ANATOMY

See Chapter 2.1, Punch Biopsy for Vulvar Lesions, Figure 2.1.1.

PATIENT POSITION

- Dorsal lithotomy on the examination table
- Colposcope positioned appropriately

LANDMARKS

- Important anatomic landmarks include the mons pubis, labia majora, labia minora, clitoris, and vaginal vestibule.
- Landmarks are principally important for documenting the site of the biopsy and the suspected pathology, based on location.

ANESTHESIA

- Local
  - Not necessary for colposcopy only.
  - For biopsy, see Chapter on Punch Biopsies for Vulvar Lesions.

EQUIPMENT

- Colposcope
- 3% to 5% acetic acid

- Procto and cotton-tip swabs
- 1% lidocaine
- 5-mL syringe
- 25-gauge, 1-1/2 inch needle
- Alcohol pads
- Sterile gauze pads
- Sterile adhesive bandage
- Tischler biopsy punch biopsy forceps or Keyes dermatologic biopsy instrument
- Adson type "pick up" forceps
- Small dissecting or iris scissors
- Formalin-filled container
- Silver nitrate or Monsel's solution

TECHNIQUE WITH ACETIC ACID

1. Liberally apply 3% to 5% acetic acid on the vulva, particularly to the suspicious-appearing areas and observe for several minutes.
2. With magnification, similar to cervical or vaginal colposcopy, abnormal areas will be raised, opaque, marginated acetowhite lesions. If such are identified, prepare for biopsy.
3. The vulva should be systematically scanned with the colposcope from the clitoris to the perineum.
4. Prep the site with chlorhexidine or isopropyl alcohol. Povidone iodine or similar, can also be used.
5. Infiltrate the biopsy site with local anesthetic. Smaller needles, for example 24 gauge or smaller will be less painful.
6. Biopsy any areas of well-demarcated, dense acetowhite lesions with or without punctuation.
7. Monsel's solution or silver nitrate can be used for hemostasis. Sutures (000 gut on a small cutting needle) are rarely needed.

CPT Codes
56820. Colposcopy of the vulva;
56821. Colposcopy of the vulva; with biopsy(s)

PEARLS

- Application of vinegar, chlorhexidine, or alcohol solutions can cause a local burning sensation and patient should be informed about this.
- A dilute epinephrine solution (1:100,000) added to the local anesthetic can reduce bleeding and reduce the amount of local necessary to get adequate anesthesia.

Bartholin's Gland Cyst/Abscess

4

Anahita Jafari, Mary Jacobson, and Paul D. Blumenthal

Bartholin's duct cysts and gland abscesses are common vulvar lesions in women of reproductive age. They result from occlusion of the duct with accumulation of mucous. They are frequently asymptomatic but accumulation of purulent material may result in the formation of a painful, rapidly enlarging, inflamed mass. In the past, Bartholin's gland abscesses were thought to mainly develop from gonorrheal or chlamydial infections. However, polymicrobial infections are also likely, and while it is still important to test for gonorrhea and chlamydia, broad-spectrum antibiotic coverage is generally recommended. Gradual involution of the Bartholin's glands can occur by 30 years of age, which may account for the higher frequency of these lesions in women between 20 and 29 years of age.

There are essentially three approaches to management of a Bartholin's cyst/abscess:

1. Simple incision and drainage, with or without the insertion of a Word catheter. A Word catheter, an inflatable bulb-tipped catheter, is typically inserted through a small stab wound into the cyst after administration of local anesthesia. The balloon is inflated with saline, and the catheter remains in place for 4 to 6 weeks. Over this time, a tract for drainage is created by epithelialization, thus providing a permanent gland opening.
2. Marsupialization. Cysts may also be opened permanently by marsupialization, in which a fistula is intentionally created by opening to the gland and suturing the cyst wall to the vulvar epithelium. This effectively prevents the duct from becoming reobstructed and causing the cyst to recur. This procedure should not be used when an abscess is present.
3. Surgical excision of the Bartholin's gland. This should be considered in patients who do not respond to conservative attempts to create a temporary or permanent drainage tract, but the procedure should only be performed when there is no active infection. Due to the potential for blood loss and deeper than expected dissection, excision is not an office-based procedure.

RELEVANT ANATOMY (Fig. 4.1)

PATIENT POSITION

- Dorsal lithotomy position

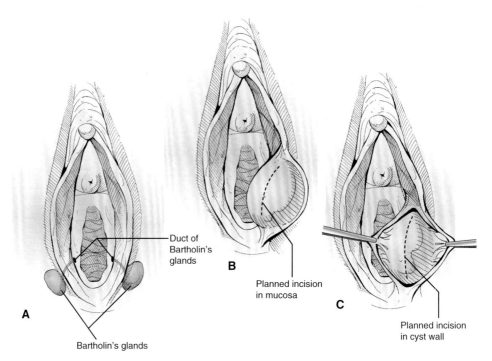

Duct of
Bartholin's
glands

Planned incision
in mucosa

Planned incision
in cyst wall

Bartholin's glands

FIGURE 4.1 ● **A:** Normal vulvar anatomy with locations of Bartholin's glands and ducts (left). **B:** Anatomic deformity of Bartholin's cyst or abscess with planned mucosal incision site (middle). **C:** Incised mucosa retracted by instruments with planned cyst wall incision site (right).

LANDMARKS

- The glands are identified bilaterally at the base of the labia minora Figure 4.1A.
- Drainage occurs through 2 to 2.5 cm-long ducts that empty into the vestibule at about the 4 o'clock and 8 o'clock positions.
- The glands are typically not palpable except in the presence of disease or infection.

ANESTHESIA

- Local anesthesia by infiltration of labial mucosa with lidocaine at planned incision site
- Intravenous narcotics or moderate sedation and analgesia may be indicated in cases of very painful lesions or for anxious patients

EQUIPMENT (Fig. 4.2)

1. Gloves
2. Sterile skin preparatory solution and drapes
3. Lidocaine, 1% or 2% solution. There is no need to use epinephrine.
4. 22–30-gauge, 1-inch needle with 5–mL syringe for injecting lidocaine
5. Scalpel blade (No. 11) and handle
6. Gauze pads (4 × 4)
7. Hemostats and sterile Q-tips
8. Culture swab

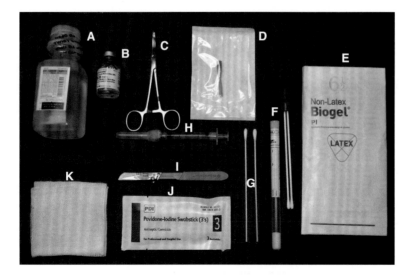

FIGURE 4.2 ● Sample instrument tray for management of Bartholin's cyst or vulvar abscess.
A: Sterile saline solution, **B:** Lidocaine, 1% or 2% solution, **C:** Hemostat, **D:** Word catheter,
E: Sterile gloves, **F:** Culture swab and transport media, **G:** Sterile Q-tips, **H:** 30-gauge, 1-inch
needle with 5–mL syringe for injecting lidocaine, **I:** Scalpel blade (No. 11) and handle, **J:** Sterile
skin preparatory solution, **K:** Gauze pads (4 × 4).

9. Sterile saline solution
10. Word catheter
11. 25-gauge, 1-inch needle with 3-mL syringe for infiltration of Word catheter bal-
    loon (not shown)

Additional Instruments for Marsupialization

- 00 absorbable suture for marsupialization
- Allis forceps

TECHNIQUE

Preparation

1. Place the patient in dorsal lithotomy position.
2. Gently separate the labia. An assistant may be helpful for retraction of the labia
   during the procedure, so that the mucosal incision site can be accessed.
3. Clean the labia and surrounding areas in the usual sterile fashion.
4. Infiltrate 2 to 3 mL of lidocaine 1% solution subcutaneously under the mucosa of
   the labium minus.

Incision and Drainage with Word Catheter Placement

1. With the No. 11 blade, make a 0.5 to 1 cm long incision into the abscess or cyst
   on the *mucosal* surface of the labium minus. The incision should be within the
   hymenal ring if possible (Fig. 4.1B).
2. Manually express the contents of the abscess sac. Use a hemostat or sterile Q-tip
   to break up loculations. The cyst contents may be sent for culture.

3. Insert the tip of the Word catheter deep into the cavity and infiltrate the balloon with 2 to 4 mL of saline. Pull slightly to insure that the balloon will not fall out of the cyst cavity.
4. Tuck the free end of the catheter into the vagina. The free end may change its position to protrude outside of the vagina. The catheter should stay in place for up to 4 weeks to allow epithelialization of the tract.
5. If a Word catheter is not used, pack the cyst cavity with iodoform gauze, ¼-inch width.

Marsupialization

1. Make a 1.5 to 3 cm (depending on size of the cyst) vertical incision in the vestibule over the center of the cyst and just outside the hymenal ring Figure 4.1C.
2. The cavity should drain spontaneously after the incision is made.
3. Grasp the cyst wall with Allis forceps and include mucosal epithelium to obtain traction and to isolate the cyst/abscess cavity.
4. The cavity may be irrigated with sterile saline, and if necessary, loculations may be broken up with a hemostat, or sterile Q-tip.
5. Evert the cyst wall and approximate to the edge of the vestibular mucosa with interrupted 00 absorbable suture. If necessary, use an Allis forceps to temporarily bind the cyst wall to the mucosa (Fig. 4.3).

AFTERCARE

• Unless there is evidence of cellulitis, antibiotic therapy is not necessary in the immunocompetent patient.
• If cellulitis is present, broad-spectrum antibiotics should be initiated before culture results are available, but the results rarely change management.

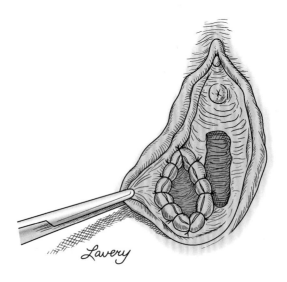

FIGURE 4.3 ● Marsupialization suture placement and final result. LifeART image copyright © 2012 Lippincott Williams & Wilkins. All rights reserved.

- All patients should be instructed to begin sitz baths 1 to 2 days post-procedure and to abstain from vaginal intercourse until the Word catheter or packing is removed.
- Analgesics may be prescribed for outpatient pain management in the initial healing period.

CPT Codes

56420.   Incision of Bartholin's Gland Cyst
56440.   Marsupialization of Bartholin's Gland Cyst

PEARLS

- When a Word catheter is not available, a simple incision and drainage with packing can be performed. Warn the patient of the high probability of abscess recurrence. Removal of the packing 2 days postprocedure is usually recommended.
- Patients older than 40 years of age should have at least a biopsy or, alternatively, complete excision of the gland to rule out Bartholin's gland cancer.
- Patients with multiple recurrences with previous treatments are candidates for definitive treatment with complete glandular excision.

Vulvar Abscess

A vulvar abscess may present as a firm, very tender, reddened, unilateral mass, which is usually the result of infectious complications of trauma or infected skin or vulvar glands.

The mass usually arises from the superior portion of the labium minus, including the clitoral hood. This is in contrast to Bartholin's cyst abscesses, which arise from the inferior portion of the labium majus (Fig. 4.1 Illustrates anatomy and deformity caused by abscess).

Many will drain spontaneously, but an incision and drainage (I&D) procedure can provide immediate relief of symptoms and definitive therapy. Typically, a simple I&D is sufficient, but broad-spectrum antibiotics are also used, especially if there is evidence of cellulitis. Findings of crepitus, dusky or necrotic tissue, or rapidly progressing erythema should raise the suspicion of necrotizing fasciitis, which will require immediate surgical intervention in the operating room.

RELEVANT ANATOMY

See Fig. 4.1A and Chapter 2.1, Punch Biopsy for Vulvar Lesions.

PATIENT POSITION

- Dorsal lithotomy position

LANDMARKS

- Vulvar abscesses are found in the labia majora or labia minora, including the clitoral hood

ANESTHESIA

- Local anesthesia by infiltration of labial epithelium with lidocaine
- Intravenous narcotics or moderate sedation and analgesia may be indicated in cases of very painful lesions or for anxious patients

EQUIPMENT (I&D) See Figure 4.2

- Gloves
- Sterile skin preparatory solution and drapes
- Ethyl chloride can also be used as a topical anesthetic
- Lidocaine, 1% or 2% solution without epinephrine
- 30-gauge, 1-inch needle with 5-mL syringe for injecting lidocaine
- Scalpel blade (No. 11) and handle
- Gauze pads (4×4)
- Hemostats and sterile Q-tips
- Culture swab
- Sterile saline solution

TECHNIQUE

Preparation

1. Place the patient in dorsal lithotomy position.
2. Clean the labia and surrounding areas in the usual sterile fashion.
3. Infiltrate 2 to 3 mL of lidocaine 1% solution subcutaneously around the edge of the abscess at either the most dependent aspect or the point with the most fluctuance.

Incision and Drainage

4. With the No. 11 blade, make a 0.5 cm long incision into the abscess.
5. Incision is made in the thinnest portion of the cyst wall, usually in the inferior, medial aspect of the mass.
6. Manually express the contents of the sac, using the hemostat or sterile Q-tip to break up loculations. The cyst contents may be sent for culture.
7. Pack the abscess cavity with ¼-inch iodoform gauze or a Word catheter.

AFTERCARE

- Broad-spectrum antibiotics should be initiated before culture results are available, but the results rarely change management.
- The gauze packing should be removed and repacked daily until the cavity can no longer be packed with the gauze. Alternatively, if a Word catheter is used it should be left in place for at least a week.
- All patients should be instructed to begin sitz baths 1 to 2 days postprocedure.
- Analgesics may be prescribed for outpatient pain management in the recovery period.

CPT Code
56405.   Incision and drainage of vulva or perineal abscess

5

Condylomata and Molluscum Contagiosum

Anahita Jafari and Paul D. Blumenthal

Destruction of Condyloma (Genital Warts)

Anogenital warts is the most common viral sexually transmitted infection in the United States. These warts, condylomata acuminata, are caused by human papilloma virus (HPV) infection, most commonly subtypes 6 and 11. The incubation period after exposure ranges from 3 weeks to 8 months. Most infections are transient and are cleared within 2 years. However, persistent infections, can be unsightly, can interfere with bodily functions such as urination and defecation, and can be socially embarrassing and ostracizing.

Treatment typically involves chemical destruction (podophyllin, 5-flourouracil, trichloroacetic acid), immunologic therapy (imiquimod, interferons, sinecatechins), or surgical excision or ablation. The choice of approach depends on location, extent of lesions, and patient preference. Medical therapies are usually tried first, and surgical therapy is generally reserved for patients with large or extensive lesions and those who have failed to respond adequately to medical therapy. Biopsy to rule out occult intraepithelial neoplasia or cancer is recommended if the lesion appears suspicious for malignancy (e.g., bleeds easily with touch, friability).

Office surgical procedures for removal of warts include cryotherapy, electrocautery, or local excision.

Colposcopic technique is sometimes useful for identifying and localizing lesions for treatment, but most lesions are visible to the naked eye.

RELEVANT ANATOMY

Generally, lesions may appear on the vulva, vagina, cervix, perineum, or anal region. Most common sites in women are the posterior introitus followed by the labia majora and labia minora. Also, external HPV infections are frequently associated with cervical lesions (Fig. 5.1).

PATIENT POSITION

• Dorsal lithotomy position

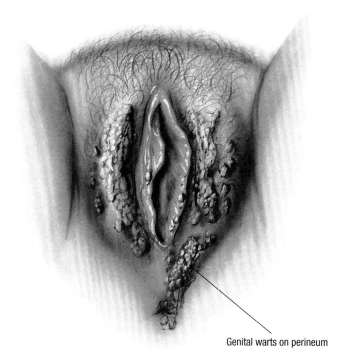

Genital warts on perineum

FIGURE 5.1 ● Genital warts (condylomata) on vulva and perineum. Asset provided by Anatomical Chart Co.

ANESTHESIA

Surgical excision and laser therapy are typically performed in an outpatient surgical suite under moderate sedation and local anesthesia, regional, or general anesthesia.

Cryotherapy, electrosurgery/dessication, and local excision may be performed in the office with local anesthesia.

Anesthesia is not required for medical treatments; however, surrounding the lesions to be treated with a layer of petroleum jelly before applying treatment, can reduce "runoff" toward anus, vagina, and other sensitive mucosal membranes.

EQUIPMENT

Graves speculum for assessing vaginal or cervical lesions

- 10% to 25% podophyllin resin in a compound with bichloro- or trichloroacetic acid
- 80% to 90% trichloroacetic acid (TCA) concentration

Cryotherapy

- Nitrous oxide units attached to a cryoprobe (use flat or needle-shaped cryotips)
- Liquid nitrogen in a fine nozzle spray gun
- Cotton-tipped swab dipped in liquid nitrogen

Electrosurgery

- Loop electrode (LEEP)
- Needle electrode (hypfercation)

Surgical Excision

- Sterile gloves
- Sterile skin preparatory solution and drapes
- Lidocaine—1% solution
- 22 to 30-gauge, 1-inch needle with 5-mL syringe for injecting lidocaine
- Scalpel blade (no. 15) and handle
- Tissue forceps
- Gauze pads (4 × 4)

4-0 absorbable suture with needle driver

TECHNIQUE

1. Review risks, benefits, and alternatives of the procedure with the patient, and obtain a written informed consent for surgical procedures.
2. Place the patient in dorsal lithotomy position.

Podophyllin Resin

- Do not use on mucosal surfaces.
- Apply to only affected areas with small cotton swab.
- Allow resin to thoroughly dry after application.
- Must be washed off within 6 hours of application.

TCA (80% to 90% Concentration)

Keratinized epithelium or mucosal surfaces

- Apply a barrier such as petroleum jelly to protect surrounding skin (Fig. 5.2).

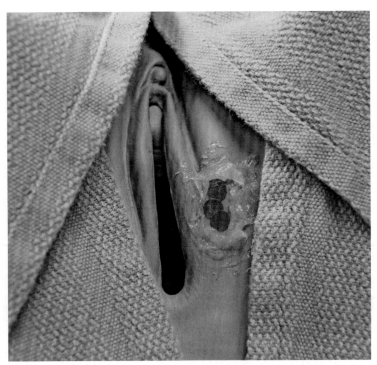

FIGURE 5.2 ● Vaseline applied around condylomata (red dots) to protect skin from application of TCA or podophyllin.

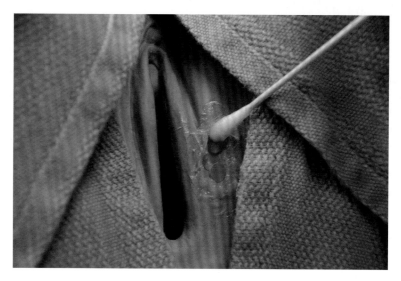

FIGURE 5.3 ● TCA being applied to condylomata (red dots) with petrolatum ointment applied to surrounding skin.

- The solution is applied directly to the lesion until it appears white or frosted (Figs. 5.3 [TCA being applied to lesion] and 5.4).
- Avoid unaffected areas adjacent to the lesion by using a small applicator such as a small cotton swab.

Cryotherapy

- Apply the cryoprobe directly to the lesion.

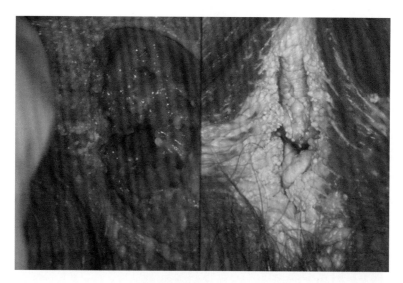

FIGURE 5.4 ● Condylomata before and after (whitening) application of acid. From Mayeaux EJ. Treatment of noncervical human papillomavirus genital infections. In: Mayeaux EJ, ed. *The essential guide to primary care procedures.* Philadelphia, PA: Lippincott Williams & Wilkins, 2009.

—or—

- Apply liquid nitrogen directly to the lesion using a cotton-tipped swab or a spray unit.
- The ice ball should extend 2 to 3 mm beyond external lesions and 5 mm beyond lesions on the cervix.
- May repeat weekly.

Electrodessication

- Clean the affected area and surroundings in normal sterile fashion.
- Apply infiltration of lidocaine 1% to the area.
- An electric needle is used to burn the lesion (Fig. 5.5).
- Scrape the burnt lesion with a small curette.
- The wound should be cleansed twice daily with hydrogen peroxide followed by an antibiotic ointment.
- Repeat treatments may be needed for recurring lesions.

Local Excision

- Clean the affected area and surroundings in normal sterile fashion.
- Infiltrate 2 to 3 mL of lidocaine 1% solution (epinephrine can be added if removing a skin lesion, to reduce bleeding) subcutaneously under the lesion (see Chapter 2.1, Punch Biopsy for Vulvar Lesions, Fig. 5.2).
- With the no. 15 blade, remove the condyloma (Fig. 5.6).
- The healthy skin edges may then be reapproximated with 1 or 2 sutures.

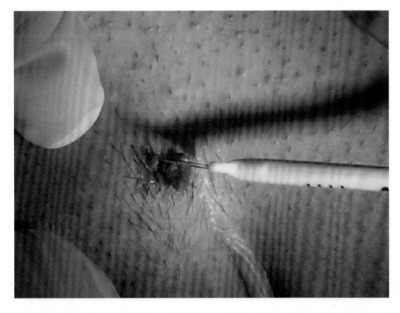

FIGURE 5.5 ● Electric needle (or loop) being applied to base of condyloma. From Mayeaux EJ. Treatment of noncervical human papillomavirus genital infections. In: Mayeaux EJ, ed. *The essential guide to primary care procedures.* Philadelphia, PA: Lippincott Williams & Wilkins, 2009.

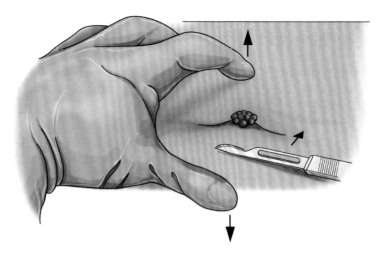

FIGURE 5.6 ● Mechanical excision of condyloma. From Mayeaux EJ. Treatment of noncervical human papillomavirus genital infections. In: Mayeaux EJ, ed. *The essential guide to primary care procedures.* Philadelphia, PA: Lippincott Williams & Wilkins, 2009.

AFTERCARE

- Meticulous postprocedure perineal hygiene is imperative to prevent superinfection.
- Pain may be treated with narcotic analgesics, but NSAIDs usually suffice.
- Topical analgesics such as lidocaine jelly may also be beneficial for some patients.

CPT Codes

56501. Destruction of lesions of the vulva, simple
56515. Destruction of lesions of the vulva, extensive
56605. Biopsy of vulva or perineum, 1 lesion
56606. Biopsy of vulva or perineum, each additional lesion

PEARLS

- Do not use podophyllin in pregnancy.
- Nitrous oxide should be avoided in the vagina and anus because of risk of fistula formation.
- Cryotherapy is safe for use during pregnancy.
- Topical 5-FU is not recommended for the treatment of external warts because of the severe inflammation, pain, and erosions experienced by the majority of patients.
- 5-FU is Category X in pregnancy.
- In general, after application of podophyllin, TCA, or imiquimod, patient can be instructed to endure the application as long as possible, then sit in a tub or similar, to wash it off.

Destruction of Molluscum Contagiosum Lesions

Molluscum contagiosum is a common, benign, viral disease of the skin and mucous membranes caused by a poxvirus. Infection and spread occurs by close bodily contact and possibly by fomites. The incubation period varies from 14 to 50 days. The individual

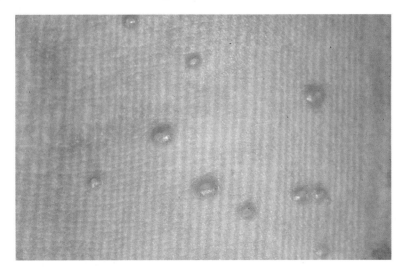

FIGURE 5.7 ● Molluscum contagiosum. Characteristic dome-shaped, shiny, waxy papules have a central white core. From Goodheart HP. *Goodheart's photoguide of common skin disorders,* 2nd ed. Philadelphia, PA: Lippincott Williams & Wilkins, 2003.

lesion is a smooth, pearly to flesh-colored, dome-shaped papule with a central umbilication. Patients with AIDS are at particular risk for infection and disseminated disease (Fig. 5.7). Characteristic dome-shaped, shiny, waxy papules have a central white core. Infection is usually self-limited and resolves spontaneously after a few months in immunocompetent individuals. Genital lesions, however, can be treated to prevent spread by sexual contact.

Treatment may consist of chemi-ablative destruction of lesions, for example, with cantharidin (applied topically), cryotherapy, or immune modulation with imiquimod. Physical interventions are also used, including electrodessication, manual extrusion of the central core by squeezing the lesion, or removal with sterilized tweezers. In the latter, sterilized tweezers are held vertically just above the skin, and the lesion is grasped and removed by gentle traction. Finally, pulsed dye lasers have shown efficacy in case reports and small, uncontrolled studies.

6

External Genitalia: Toluidine Blue Testing in Victims of Sexual Assault/Abuse

Katharine Anne Willoughby and Harise Stein

Typical patterns of genital trauma can often be seen in victims of nonconsensual intercourse. The most common injury noted is linear tears to the posterior four-chette. The use of toluidine blue, a dye that preferentially stains exposed to super-ficial nuclei, may enhance the ability to detect subtle trauma. The interpretation of these results can at times be confusing, since consensual intercourse may also cause similar findings. However, it is the responsibility of the physician to collect all available data and then allow the court to determine its significance in each individual case.

RELEVANT ANATOMY (Fig. 6.1)

PATIENT POSITION

- Dorsal lithotomy
- Consider prone knee-chest for children

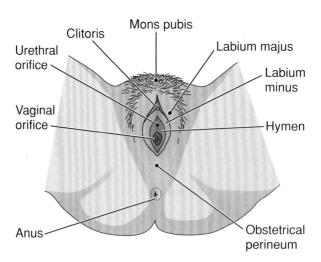

FIGURE 6.1 ● External genitalia with perineum. From Cohen BJ, Taylor JJ. *Memmler's the human body in health and disease,* 10th ed. Baltimore, MD: Lippincott Williams & Wilkins, 2005.

LANDMARKS

- None

ANESTHESIA

- None
- May require examination under anesthesia for children

EQUIPMENT

- 1% aqueous solution toluidine blue
- Cotton-tipped swabs
- Water-based lubricating jelly
- Cotton balls
- Colposcope (optional but recommended)
- Digital camera (optional but recommended)

TECHNIQUE

1. Place the patient in the dorsal lithotomy position.
2. Prior to digital or speculum examination, which might cause additional tissue injury, carefully visually inspect the external genitalia unaided and then with the colposcope.
3. Record any areas of:
   a. "TEARS" (i.e., Tears, Ecchymoses, Abrasions, Redness, and Swelling) (Figs. 6.2, 6.3)
   b. Inflammation, discharge, atrophy

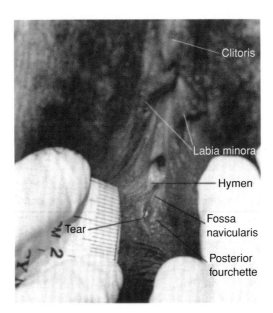

FIGURE 6.2 ● Tear to posterior fourchette. Female Tanner 4 sexual assault patient. From Olshaker JS, Jackson MC, Smock WS, eds. *Forensic emergency medicine,* 2nd ed. Philadelphia, PA: Lippincott Williams & Wilkins, 2007.

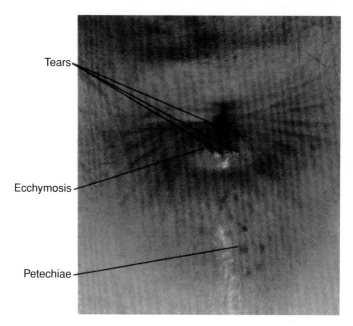

Tears

Ecchymosis

Petechiae

FIGURE 6.3 ● Anal trauma in a female with a history of anal penetration. From Olshaker JS, Jackson MC, Smock WS, eds. *Forensic emergency medicine,* 2nd ed. Philadelphia, PA: Lippincott Williams & Wilkins, 2007.

4. Apply the toluidine blue stain with cotton-tipped swabs to the perineum and perianal areas, with particular attention to the posterior fourchette, hymen, labia minora, and anus. Allow the stain to dry for a few seconds.
5. Gently wipe away the stain with a cotton ball moistened with lubricating jelly. Continue wiping the area with fresh cotton balls until no further stain is recovered. A dry cotton-tipped swab may be used to gently remove dye from fine creases. The dye will be retained at sites of injury.
6. A colposcope may be used to further examine dyed areas.
7. Document all areas of staining with toluidine blue. Photographs may also be taken to be used later as evidence.

AFTERCARE

• None

CPT Code: 99285—Emergency department visit for the evaluation and management of a patient, which requires these three key components within the constraints imposed by the urgency of the patient's clinical condition and/or mental status: A comprehensive history; a comprehensive examination; and medical decision making of high complexity. Counseling and/or coordination of care with other providers or agencies is provided consistent with the nature of the problem(s) and the patient's and/or family's needs. Usually, the presenting problem(s) are of high severity and pose an immediate significant threat to life or physiologic function.

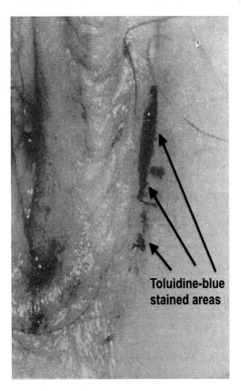

Toluidine-blue stained areas

FIGURE 6.4 ● Excess toluidine pooling in folds. From Dirnhofer R. Effects of toluidine blue and destaining reagents used in sexual assault examinations on the ability to obtain DNA profiles from postcoital vaginal swabs. *J Forensic Sci* 1997;42(2):316–319.

PEARLS

- Multiple factors impact the likelihood that trauma will be found at the time of examination, including time lapse since the alleged trauma, age, skin color, parity, and history of prior sexual activity.
- Inflammation or infection may lead to patchy uptake of toluidine blue; correlate with prior visual inspection.
- Excess toluidine may pool increases and mimics the linear uptake seen in trauma (Fig. 6.4); be sure to remove all excess.

Vaginal Swab Testing for GC/CT in Teens—Self-Testing and Clinician Testing

Katharine Anne Willoughby and Paula J. A. Hillard

Adolescent females as a group have historically had the highest rates of *Neisseria gonorrhoeae* and *Chlamydia trachomatis* infection of any age group. However, discomfort associated with the gynecologic speculum examination and endocervical specimen collection may limit rates of screening. Alternatively, vaginal swab collection, either performed by a practitioner or the patient, is an effective, well-tolerated method of screening. Urine-based nucleic acid amplification testing (NAAT) is also being used extensively in asymptomatic adolescent populations.

RELEVANT ANATOMY

- Endocervical (NOT vaginal) clinician testing
- Vaginal self-swab

PATIENT POSITION

- Variable
  - Dorsal lithotomy may be used for practitioner collection
  - Patient may choose position if performing self-collection (squatting, sitting on toilet, standing with one foot on toilet or stool)

LANDMARKS

- None

ANESTHESIA

- None

EQUIPMENT

- Amplified DNA probe collection/transport kit.
- Alternatively, testing for gonorrhea and chlamydia can be performed on urine samples utilizing NAAT technology.

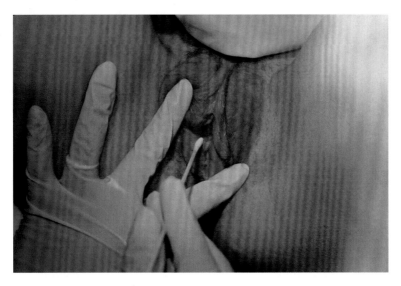

FIGURE 7.1.1 ● Dacron-tipped swab being inserted into vagina. From Sweet RL, Gibbs RS. *Atlas of infectious diseases of the female genital tract.* Philadelphia, PA: Lippincott Williams & Wilkins, 2005.

TECHNIQUE

1. Clinician testing, endocervical. Recommended in adolescents with symptomatic discharge or those tolerant of pelvic examination.
   a. Assist patient into the dorsal lithotomy position on the gynecologic examination table.
   b. Insert speculum into vagina (Pederson or Huffman speculum preferable for most adolescents).
   c. Swab cervix with large cotton swab (supplied with collection kit) to remove mucous and secretions.
   d. Insert the Dacron-tipped swab that is supplied with the collection kit 1 inch into the endocervix.
   e. Rotate the swab 360 degrees twice and leave in place for the time recommended by the manufacturer.
   f. Place the swab in the collection container.
2. Clinician testing, vaginal. This method may be used if the patient declines speculum examinations but prefers clinician to collect specimen.
   a. Assist patient into the dorsal lithotomy position on the gynecologic examination table.
   b. Insert the Dacron-tipped swab that is supplied with the collection kit 1 inch into the vagina (Fig. 7.1.1).
   c. Leave in place for the time recommended by the manufacturer.
   d. Place the swab in the collection container.
3. Self-testing. Preferred method for patients who are uncomfortable with clinician performing collection.
   a. The patient is instructed to insert the Dacron-tipped swab that is supplied with the collection kit 1 inch into the vagina, leaving it in place for the time recommended by the manufacturer.

AFTERCARE

• None

CPT Codes
87486. Chlamydia probe nucleic acid testing amplification
87081. Culture, screening

PEARLS

• Clinician testing is preferable in symptomatic females. However, adolescents who decline a pelvic examination should be screened with either self-collected specimens or with urine-based NAAT.
• A patient's preference for clinician versus self-swab collection is dependent on many factors, including the patient's trust in the individual clinician.

Wet Prep and Potassium Hydroxide for Assessing Vaginitis

Katharine Anne Willoughby and Paula J. A. Hillard

Vulvovaginitis is a common presenting complaint. Three common causes, bacterial vaginosis, trichomoniasis, and candidiasis, can quickly and easily be diagnosed by performing a wet prep—a microscopic examination of vaginal secretions in the office. However, the sensitivity of this testing is less than that of culture, and it varies among these common diagnoses. The wet prep is typically performed in conjunction with a potassium hydroxide (KOH) prep to look for vaginal candidiasis. KOH selectively lyses epithelial cells, as well as red and white blood cells, making it easier to identify unaffected fungal elements if present.

RELEVANT ANATOMY

The various organisms causing vulvovaginitis infect different areas of the female anatomy. Trichomonas is a vaginal pathogen, while Candida infects both the vagina and vulva.

PATIENT POSITION

- Dorsal lithotomy

LANDMARKS

- Wet prep specimen is optimally taken from the anterior vaginal fornix, as the posterior fornix is more likely to be contaminated by semen or vaginally applied medications.

ANESTHESIA

- None

EQUIPMENT (Fig. 7.2.1)

- Speculum
- pH tape
- Cotton-tipped swab

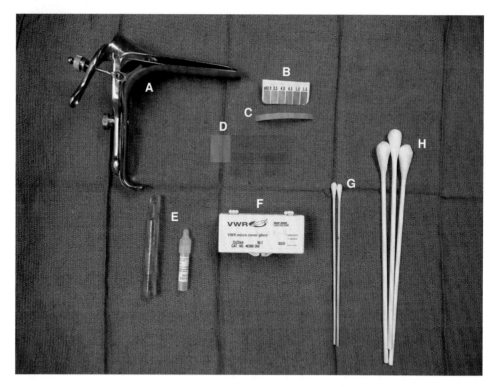

FIGURE 7.2.1 ● Wet prep/mount tray. **A:** Graves or Pederson speculum, **B:** pH paper scale, **C:** pH tape, **D:** Frosted slide, **E:** Saline and KOH solution, **F:** Cover slips, **G:** Q-tip, and **H:** Procto swabs.

- Glass slide(s)
- Cover slip (2)
- 0.9% saline (1 to 2 drops)
- 10% KOH (1 to 2 drops)
- Microscope

TECHNIQUE

1. Place the patient in the dorsal lithotomy position.
2. Insert the speculum. Make note of any discharge, purulence, or erythema of the vulva, vagina, or cervix (Fig. 7.2.2).
3. Apply a strip of pH paper to the vaginal side wall. Avoid the posterior fornix, as blood, semen, or cervical mucus can alter result. A pH above 4.5 in a premenopausal woman suggests bacterial vaginosis or trichomoniasis, while a pH of 4 to 4.5 suggests Candidal infection.
4. Place two drops of normal saline on one end of glass slide, typically the frosted end, and one drop of 10% KOH at the other (alternatively, two slides can be used).
5. Collect a sample of vaginal discharge on a cotton-tipped swab and transfer first to the drop of saline, and then to the drop of KOH.
6. Examine slides under microscope with both low- and high-power magnification. Note any clue cells or motile trichomonads present on the slide prepared with normal saline, and any hyphae noted on the slide prepared with KOH.

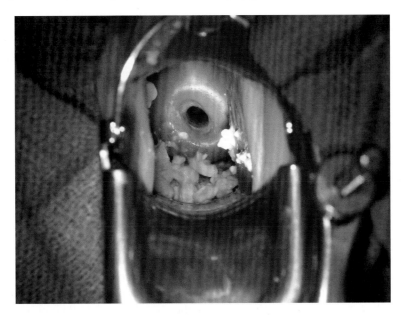

FIGURE 7.2.2   ●   "Cottage Cheese" discharge visible in vaginal vault.

AFTERCARE

• None

CPT Code

87210.   Smear, primary source with interpretation; wet mount for infectious agents (e.g., saline, India ink, KOH preps)

PEARLS

• Classically, trichomoniasis is associated with a greenish-yellow frothy discharge, although many infections are asymptomatic.
• Bacterial vaginosis may associated with a "fishy"-smelling thin discharge that is accentuated when KOH is applied to the specimen, and candidiasis is associated with a white, thick, "cottage cheese" discharge. However, the appearance of the discharge alone is not reliable for diagnosis, and a wet prep and KOH should be performed routinely.
• Since bacterial vaginosis does not cause inflammation, white blood cells (WBCs) typically are not seen. The presence of WBCs suggests candidiasis, trichomoniasis, or a cervicitis.
• Sexually transmitted infection (STI) testing should be performed in addition to a wet prep in individuals at risk for STIs, as symptoms can be similar.
• Wet prep is only 50% to 66% sensitive for the detection of trichomoniasis, 50% to 80% sensitive for candidiasis, and 80% to 85% sensitive for bacterial vaginosis when compared to culture. If clinical suspicion is high in the context of a negative wet prep, cultures, rapid antigen detection testing, or nucleic acid amplification testing (NAAT) should be employed.

Vaginal Cultures

Katharine Anne Willoughby and
Paula J. A. Hillard

The etiology of vaginitis cannot always be determined by history, physical, and wet prep. When a diagnosis remains unclear, a vaginal culture should be performed. Cultures have long been held as the gold standard for detection of trichomoniasis, and cultures have significantly improved detection rates for candidiasis as opposed to wet prep. When a diagnosis is not clear or when there is evidence of cervicitis on examination, cervical testing for STIs is indicated.

Vaginal cultures are commonly used in pregnancy for the detection of Group B Streptococcus at approximately 36 weeks of gestation.

Other specific bacterial pathogens are uncommon; Group A Streptococcus may be seen in breastfeeding women, children, or those with atrophic vaginas.

RELEVANT ANATOMY

Trichomonas is a vaginal pathogen, while candida may infect both the vagina and vulva.

PATIENT POSITION

- Dorsal lithotomy

LANDMARKS

- None

ANESTHESIA

- None

EQUIPMENT

- Speculum.
- Fungal culture collection kit or PCR detection kit (for suspected candidal infection). Specimen may require immediate plating on agar plates.
- Amplified DNA probe or NAAT collection/transport kit (for suspected cervicitis).
- Culture collection kit, amplified RNA test, or NAAT (for suspected trichomoniasis).

TECHNIQUE

1. Place the patient in the dorsal lithotomy position.
2. Place the speculum and adjust to achieve visualization of the cervix.
3. If a candidal infection is suspected, swab the vaginal walls or the affected area with the swab provided with the fungal culture kit. Place the swab in the provided collection container or plate on agar, as required by your laboratory.
4. If a cervicitis is suspected (Figs. 7.3.1, 7.3.2), remove the excess cervical mucus from the cervical os with the cotton-tipped swab provided in the collection kit. Place the Dacron-tipped swab within the endocervical canal and rotate 360 degrees twice and leave in place for the amount of time recommended by the manufacturer. Remove swab and place within the provided transport medium.

AFTERCARE

- Await results of cultures before treating.

CPT Code

87210. Smear, primary source with interpretation; wet mount for infectious agents (e.g., saline, India ink, KOH preps)

PEARLS

- While culture remains the gold standard for diagnosing gonorrhea and chlamydia infections, this method has largely been replaced with nucleic acid amplification tests (NAAT) which have better sensitivity and specificity.
- Vaginal cultures are not indicated when findings suggest bacterial vaginosis. The presence on culture of Gardnerella vaginale does not indicate bacterial vaginosis.

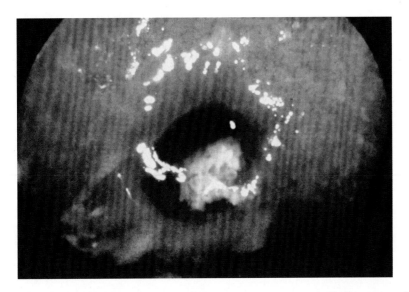

FIGURE 7.3.1 ● Chlamydial mucopurulent cervicitis. From Sweet RL, Gibbs RS. *Atlas of infectious diseases of the female genital tract.* Philadelphia, PA: Lippincott Williams & Wilkins, 2005.

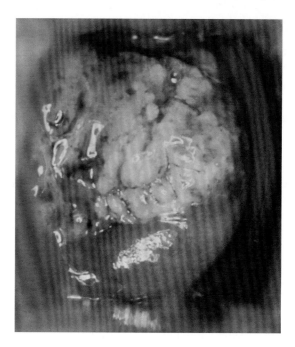

FIGURE 7.3.2 ● Herpes simplex cervicitis. From Sweet RL, Gibbs RS. *Atlas of infectious diseases of the female genital tract.* Philadelphia, PA: Lippincott Williams & Wilkins, 2005.

- Infection with trichomonas is more common in many adolescent populations than gonorrhea. Wet prep has poor sensitivity for this pathogen, while culture is held as the gold standard.
- Culture is the gold standard for diagnosing yeast vaginitis.

8

Colposcopy: Vagina and Cervix

Inna Landres and Paul D. Blumenthal

Colposcopy is a diagnostic procedure used to magnify the cervix and vagina and assess for premalignant or malignant epithelial changes. Indications for cervical colposcopy are abnormal cytology results from a screening pap smear including atypical squamous cells-uncertain significance (ASC-US) with high-risk human papilloma virus (HPV) subtype, low-grade squamous intraepithelial lesion (LSIL), high-grade squamous intraepithelial lesion (HSIL), ASC suggestive of high-grade lesion (ASC-H), atypical glandular cells (AGC), or results suspicious for invasive cancer. Indications for vaginal colposcopy include vaginal intraepithelial neoplasia (VAIN) on vaginal screening pap or abnormalities noted on physical examination.

RELEVANT ANATOMY

Cervix and vagina are the anatomical targets for this procedure. For satisfactory colposcopy of the cervix in particular, the operator must obtain an unobstructed view of the cervix and must have room to manipulate it in order to obtain the necessary visualization.

PATIENT POSITION

Gynecologic examination table in a dorsal lithotomy position

LANDMARKS (Fig. 8.1)

- Transformation zone
- Squamocolumnar junction
- Endocervix
- Ectocervix

ANESTHESIA

- Typically none; may offer paracervical block if extensive biopsies are taken.
- Lidocaine gel or similar may also be applied to cervix in advance of biopsy.

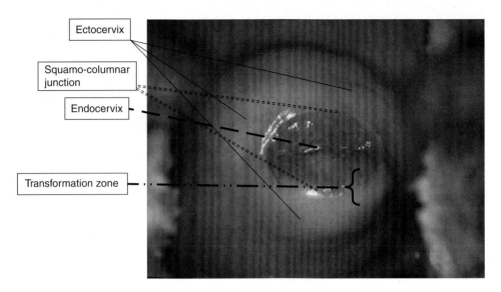

Ectocervix

Squamo-columnar junction

Endocervix

Transformation zone

FIGURE 8.1 ● Colposcopic landmarks.

EQUIPMENT

- Colposcope or other digital or video imaging device
- Speculum
- Endocervical speculum for visualization into the canal
- 3% acetic acid solution
- Cotton-tip applicator/Q tips
- Lugol's iodine solution
- Biopsy forceps
  - Tischler or Kevorkian are most common types
  - Stiff brush (Spirabrush is a recent innovation)
- Cytobrush
- Endocervical curette
  - Kevorkian with open or grated basket
- Silver nitrite
- Monsel's solution
- Dedicated form for documenting and mapping colposcopic results

TECHNIQUE

   I. Colposcopy
1. Insert a Graves speculum into vagina and obtain unobstructed view of cervix.
2. Remove any mucus, blood, or discharge that obscures visualization using a cotton Q tip soaked in saline.
3. Examine the cervix and vagina grossly under bright light for any obvious areas of erosion, ulceration, or leukoplakia.
4. Apply 3% acetic acid solution liberally to the cervix with cotton swabs for up to 60 seconds.

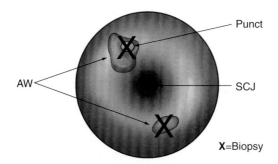

FIGURE 8.2 ● Record abnormal lesions and biopsy sites. From Thomas J. Zuber, EJ. Mayeaux Jr. *Atlas of primary care procedures.* Philadelphia, PA: Lippincott Williams & Wilkins, 2004.

5. Identify the transformation zone circumferentially around the cervical os, using endocervical speculum, if necessary.
   a. Satisfactory: Adequate visualization of the entire transformation zone
   b. Unsatisfactory: Inability to visualize the transformation zone or only partial visualization
6. Note any areas of acetowhite changes or abnormal vascularity and record the distribution by dividing the cervix as a clock (Fig. 8.2).
   a. Evaluate for patterns such as punctation, mosaicism, or abnormal appearing vessels that suggest moderate or severe dysplasia.
   b. Draw a map of any lesions noted and their location, using the face of the cervix as a clock, with the cervical os at the center, and the squamocolumnar junction drawn as it appears on the ectocervix for reference.
   c. Consider digital photography and save for medical records (if available).
7. Use the green filter examination to accentuate any abnormal vasculature.
8. Dilute Lugol's iodine solution may be used to aid in detection (Schiller's test).
9. Obtain biopsies from any concerning areas, label and place biopsies in formalin (Figs. 8.2 and 8.3).
   a. Sensitivity can be improved by performing a biopsy in each quadrant, but unless a very small biopsy instrument is used, it can also increase bleeding and discomfort.
10. Perform Endocervical Curettage (ECC) for AGC, ASC-H, HSIL, adenocarcinoma in situ (AIS), and for unsatisfactory colposcopy (For women <25 years old, with "inadequate colposcopy" and for whom only low grade cytology or ASC-US was the indication for colposcopy, repeat tesing at 6-months is preferable to ECC).
    a. Introduce the endocervical curette up to the internal os and rotate to scrape all four quadrants (Fig. 8.4).
    b. Use an endocervical cytobrush to remove any exfoliated tissue.
II. Vaginal Colposcopy
   1. Apply 3% acetic acid solution liberally to the vagina.
   2. Examine the vagina systematically and straighten out any folds and rugae by opening the speculum, rotate the speculum to examine anterior and posterior vagina.
   3. Biopsy any suspicious vaginal lesions.

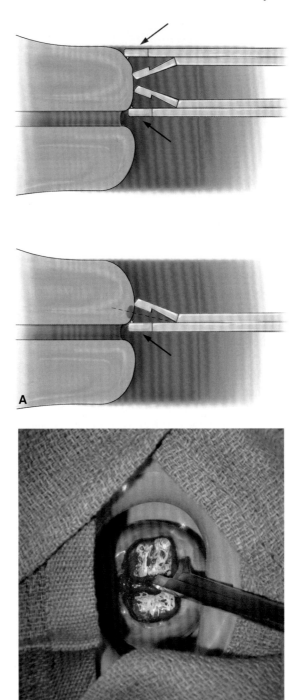

FIGURE 8.3 ● Performing a cervical biopsy. **A:** Orientation of biopsy forceps on exocervix. From Thomas J. Zuber, EJ. Mayeaux Jr. *Atlas of primary care procedures.* Philadelphia, PA: Lippincott Williams & Wilkins, 2004. **B:** Biopsy forceps placed against cervical lesion (original photo).

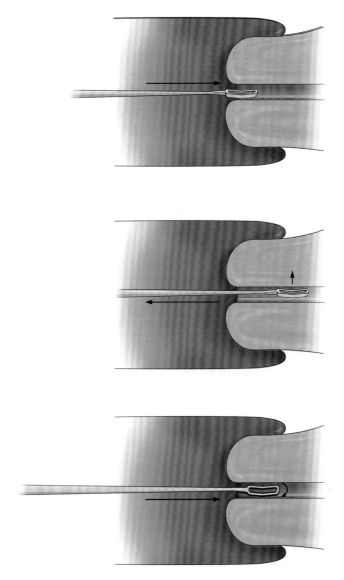

FIGURE 8.4 ● Performing ECC. From Thomas J. Zuber, EJ. Mayeaux Jr. *Atlas of primary care procedures.* Philadelphia, PA: Lippincott Williams & Wilkins, 2004.

III. Colposcopy in pregnant patients
    1. Avoid ECC.
    2. Limit biopsies to lesions suggesting *severe* dysplasia or invasive cancer.
    3. Anticipate heavier bleeding if biopsies are obtained.
    4. Schedule postpartum follow-up for repeat colposcopy.

AFTERCARE

- Bleeding from biopsy sites
  - Apply direct pressure.
  - Silver nitrite—Dry area with cotton swab and then immediately apply silver nitrate stick.
  - Monsel's solution—Apply liberally to bleeding area and observe for styptic effect.

- Patient instructions
  - Avoid intercourse and tampons for 1 week to minimize bleeding and trauma.
  - May notice spotting and dark-colored discharge from application of Monsel's, similar to coffee grounds-colored discharge.
  - Contact office if any excessive bleeding, fever, or pain.

CPT Codes
56820. **Colposcopy** of the vulva
56821. **Colposcopy** of the vulva; with biopsy(s)
57420. **Colposcopy** of the entire vagina, with cervix if present
57421. **Colposcopy** of the entire vagina, with cervix if present; with biopsy(s) of vagina/cervix
57452. **Colposcopy** of the cervix including upper/adjacent vagina
57454. **Colposcopy** of the cervix including upper/adjacent vagina; with biopsy(s) of the cervix and ECC
57455. **Colposcopy** of the cervix including upper/adjacent vagina; with biopsy(s) of the cervix
57456. **Colposcopy** of the cervix including upper/adjacent vagina; with ECC
57460. **Colposcopy** of the cervix including upper/adjacent vagina; with loop electrode biopsy(s) of the cervix
57461. **Colposcopy** of the cervix including upper/adjacent vagina; with loop electrode conization of the cervix

PEARLS

- Use a spray bottle of 3% acetic acid for colposcopy of vagina, but insure liberal application.
- Use a condom with the end cut off around the speculum when redundant vaginal walls obscure visualization of the cervix.

9

Imperforate Hymen, Hymenotomy, and Division of the Hymenal Band

Kevin Henry Maas and Paula J. A.Hillard

Imperforate hymen occurs as a result of the failure of the hymen to canalize during the perinatal period, and occurs within incidence of approximately 1 in 1,000. Hymenal variants, including microperforate hymen, hymenal bands, cribriform hymen, or high navicular hymen are more common than imperforate hymen. The differential diagnosis for imperforate hymen includes vaginal agenesis (Mayer–Rokitansky–Kuster–Hauser syndrome), a distal transverse vaginal septum, and androgen insensitivity syndrome (AIS). Diagnosis MUST be established before treatment is undertaken to avoid inadvertently operating on one of these conditions without appropriate surgical planning.

Symptomatic Imperforate Hymen in the Neonate (Fig. 9.1)

- THIS IS NOT AN OFFICE PROCEDURE.
- Imperforate hymen may present in the neonatal period as either hydrocolpos or mucocolpos, secondary to maternal estradiol stimulation of the neonatal vaginal epithelium.
- Hydro/mucocolpos presents in the newborn as a translucent, bulging yellow-gray mass at the vaginal introitus (Fig. 9.1).
- They are typically asymptomatic and spontaneously resolve. However, large hydro/mucocolpos has the potential to obstruct the ureters, resulting in hydronephrosis. Diagnosis must be well established before surgery, as other genitourinary anomalies may be associated. Hymenotomy should be performed under general anesthesia in these circumstances.

Asymptomatic Imperforate Hymen in Childhood

- THIS IS NOT AN OFFICE PROCEDURE.
- Asymptomatic girls should be monitored through childhood.
- The optimal time for hymenotomy in these patients is after the onset of thelarche, but before menarche.
- Differential diagnoses should be considered with imaging performed after the onset of puberty with ultrasound and/or MRI.

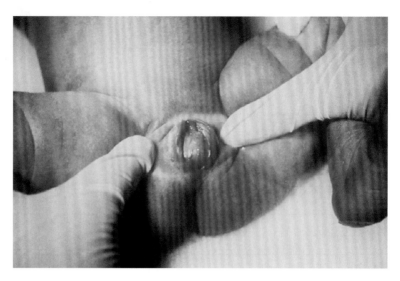

FIGURE 9.1 ● Imperforate hymen in the neonate. Used with permission from Emans SJ, Laufer MR, Goldstein DP, eds. *Pediatric and adolescent gynecology.* 5th ed. Philadelphia, PA: Lippincott Williams & Wilkins; 2005:plate 21.

Hematocolpos (Fig. 9.2)

- THIS IS NOT AN OFFICE PROCEDURE.
- The most common presentation of imperforate hymen is cyclic or persistent pelvic pain during puberty.

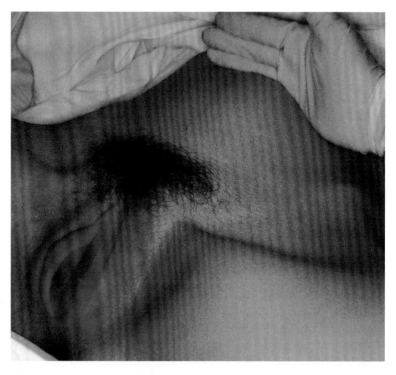

FIGURE 9.2 ● Palpation of the abdomen in this 14-year-old girl revealed a distended uterus, rising to the level of the umbilicus. From Fleisher GR, Ludwig S, Baskin MN. *Atlas of pediatric emergency medicine.* Philadelphia, PA: Lippincott Williams & Wilkins, 2004.

- Hematocolpos presents as a translucent blue-tinged bulge at the perineum.
- Hymenotomy should be performed under general anesthesia to remove obstruction and provide symptomatic relief.

Hymenal Variants—Hymenal Bands (Fig. 9.3)

- Hymenal bands or other hymenal variants may rarely present with recurrent UTIs in childhood, but more frequently preclude tampon use after menarche or prevent intercourse.
- If or when desired, and if an examination and hymenal manipulation are tolerated by an adolescent in the office, some of these variants may be treated in the office.
- More frequently, an examination is NOT tolerated, and the procedure should be performed with general anesthesia.

RELEVANT ANATOMY (Figs. 9.3 and 9.4)

PATIENT POSITION

- Patient is placed in the dorsal lithotomy position.

LANDMARKS (Fig. 9.4)

- Hymenal ring
- Urethra
- Anus

ANESTHESIA

- Hymenotomy is generally performed as a same-day surgery under general anesthesia.
- If a **hymenal band** is to be excised in the office, infiltration with 1% lidocaine is appropriate.

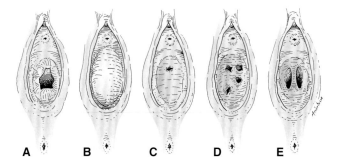

FIGURE 9.3 ● Hymenal Variants (**A**) normal, (**B**) imperforate, (**C**) microperforate, (**D**) cribriform, and (**E**) septate. Used with permission from Emans SJ, Laufer MR, Goldstein DP, eds. *Pediatric and adolescent gynecology.* 5th ed. Philadelphia, PA: Lippincott Williams & Wilkins, 2005:10.

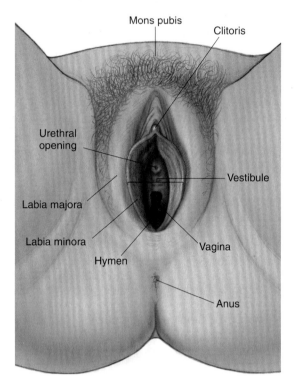

FIGURE 9.4 ● The female external genitalia—inferior view. From Westheimer R, Lopater S. *Human sexuality.* Baltimore, MD: Lippincott Williams & Wilkins, 2003.

EQUIPMENT (for in-office division of hymenal band)

- 2% lidocaine jelly
- 1% lidocaine for injection—without epinephrine
- 3-0 or 4-0 delayed absorbable sutures
- Hemostat
- Fine tissue scissors (e.g., iris scissors)
- Suture scissors

TECHNIQUE (for division of hymenal band)

1. Patient is asked to void and places feet in stirrups of examination table.
2. 2% lidocaine jelly is placed at the hymenal ring to allow an adequate examination and assessment to confirm the diagnosis of hymenal band (vs. vaginal septum)
3. 1% lidocaine is injected into hymenal band.
4. Hemostat is placed behind the band (Fig. 9.5).
5. Two ~10-inch lengths of suture are placed behind the band.
6. One suture is tied anterior on the band, and the second is tied posterior, leaving distance between the two-tied sutures.
7. Hymenal band is cut using tissue scissors.
8. Suture is trimmed.

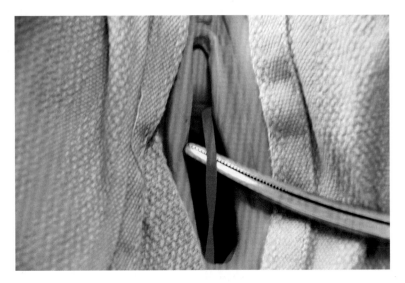

FIGURE 9.5 ● Hemostat placed behind hymenal band prior to ligation and excision.

AFTERCARE

- Postoperative pain is typically minimal, but a prescription for topical 2% lidocaine jelly should be provided. Use prior to urination is helpful.
- Sitz baths further assist with healing.

CPT Codes
    56442. **Hymenotomy,** simple incision
           OR
    56700. Partial hymenectomy or revision of hymenal ring
           OR
    56501. Destruction of lesion(s), vulva; simple (e.g., electrosurgery, if cautery alone would suffice.

PEARLS

- Any hymenal variation other than a single, thin, hymenal band most frequently warrants excision with adequate general anesthesia in a surgical center or operating room.
- Diagnosis of imperforate hymen MUST be established prior to attempted incision, as other genital anomalies require careful planning and different surgical techniques, and should be performed by a gynecologist skilled in managing genital anomalies and addressing the medical, psychosocial, and psychosexual needs of adolescents.
- The use of knee crutches (as opposed to conventional stirrups) can increase patient comfort and ability to relax.

10

Pudendal Block

Stephanie Gustin and Paul D. Blumenthal

Most commonly used for perineal anesthesia prior to episiotomy or repair of perineal tears at delivery, the pudendal block has also demonstrated efficacy in treating conditions such as pudendal neuralgia, vulvodynia, and vulvar vestibulitis, as well as providing anesthesia for minor perineal office gynecologic procedures. The pudendal nerve arises from the S2, S3, and S4 nerve roots (Fig. 10.1). The nerve leaves the pelvis via the greater sciatic foramen. It courses beneath the ischial spine, just medial to the internal pudendal artery. The pudendal nerve then reenters the pelvis by way of Alcock's canal, where it splits into its three terminal branches: The inferior hemorrhoidal, deep perineal, and superficial perineal nerves.

RELEVANT ANATOMY

- The target is the pudendal nerve as it traverses through the lesser sciatic notch (Fig. 10.1).
- Successful blockade may be achieved via a transcutaneous (perineal) or transvaginal approach; both will be described.
- Note: We recommend the use of a needle guide (trumpet) when attempting the transvaginal approach in order to protect the provider from unintended needle sticks, and the woman from unintended vaginal trauma during the vaginal approach to the sciatic notch.

PATIENT POSITION

- Lithotomy

LANDMARKS

- Ischial spine and ischial tuberosity for the transvaginal and transgluteal approaches, respectively.

EQUIPMENT

Transvaginal Approach

- Gloves
- 30 mL of 1% lidocaine or similar amount of 0.5% Bupivacaine
- 10- to 20-mL syringe with finger and thumbholes
- Iowa Trumpet kit

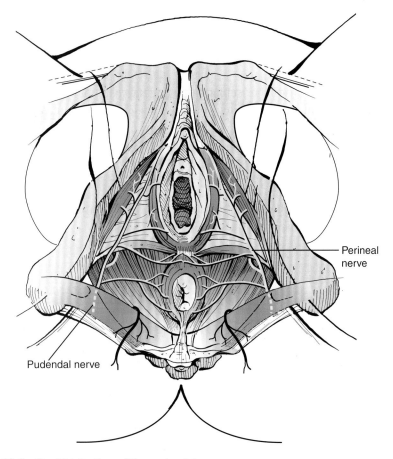

FIGURE 10.1 ● Distribution of the pudendal nerve.

- Prepackaged kits usually contain both the trumpet and needle and a syringe pre-filled with drug.
- If a kit is unavailable, a 15-cm, 22-gauge needle may be used cautiously.

Transgluteal Approach

- Gloves
- 30 mL of 1% lidocaine or 0.5% Bupivacaine
- 10- to 20-mL syringe with finger and thumbholes
- 15-cm, 22-gauge needle

TECHNIQUE

Transvaginal Approach (Fig. 10.2)

1. Open the Iowa Trumpet kit and put on gloves.
2. Beginning on the patient's left side, place the left index and middle fingers into the vagina.
3. Palpate deep, posteriorly, and laterally, in attempts to locate the ischial spine.
   a. The ischial spine is a bony prominence that feels separate from the pelvic sidewall.

4. Once the ischial spine has been located, the sacrospinous ligament, connecting the ischial spine to the sacrum, can be palpated as a thick band running in a medial and posterior direction.
   a. The pudendal nerve is located just medial to the ischial spine, and inferior to the sacrospinous ligament.
5. Upon identification of the ischial spine and sacrospinous ligament, guide the trumpet (without needle) using your right hand along your vaginally placed fingers.
   a. Confirm that the trumpet is placed just medial and posterior to the ischial spine, along the sacrospinous ligament.
6. Once the trumpet is aligned, slide the needle along the trumpet until completely placed.
   a. The tip of the needle should extend 10 mm from the trumpet, thus perforating through the sacrospinous ligament (Fig. 10.2, **inset**)

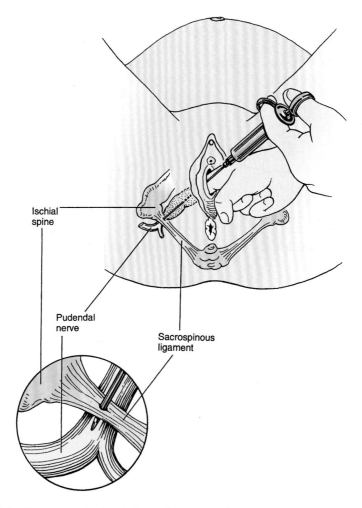

Ischial spine

Pudendal nerve

Sacrospinous ligament

FIGURE 10.2 ● Transvaginal technique. Illustration of locating the landmarks. Inset: Trumpet in place in relation to landmarks. From Beckmann CRB, Ling FW, Laube DW, et al. *Obstetrics and gynecology,* 4th ed. Baltimore, MD: Lippincott Williams & Wilkins, 2002.

7. Take care to aspirate (pull back on the plunger) to confirm that you have not entered a vessel.
   a. If blood is returned via aspiration, carefully withdraw the needle, recheck your position, and make another attempt.
   b. Never inject if blood is aspirated.
8. Inject 10 mL of 1% lidocaine.
9. Repeat the procedure on the right side.
10. Once both sides have been injected, wait at least 2 minutes and then test the area using forceps. If sensation is intact, wait an additional 2 minutes and then retest.

Transcutaneous (Fig. 10.3)

1. Palpate the left ischial tuberosity through the buttock (Fig. 10.3).
2. Once identified, transgluteally introduce the 15-cm, 22-gauge needle aiming just medial to the spine. The needle should penetrate to approximately 2.5 cm.
3. Aspirate, and then inject 8 to 10 mL of lidocaine.
4. Repeat on the right side.
5. Additional lidocaine may be directed to deep and superficial tissue of the vulva, anteriorly, to block the ilioinguinal and genitofemoral nerves, if desired.
6. Test the perineum for anesthetic effect as for the transvaginal approach.

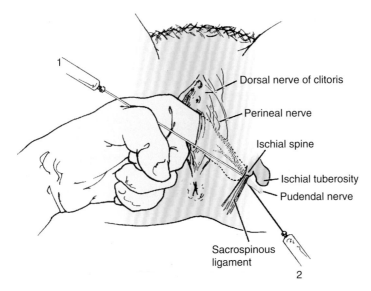

FIGURE 10.3 ● Transcutaneous/perineal approach to a pudendal block. **1.** Transvaginal approach, **2.** Transgluteal approach. From Snell. *Clinical anatomy,* 7th ed. Lippincott Williams & Wilkins, 2003.

AFTERCARE

- Patient to observe for possible swelling and pressure in perineal area as a result of possible compromise of or injury to pudendal vessels.

CPT Code

64430.   Injection, anesthetic agent; pudendal nerve

PEARLS

- Allow appropriate time for the block, as failure to wait a sufficient amount of time is a common cause of failure of pudendal blocks.
- Make sure to aspirate frequently during administration of local anesthetic, as the pudendal nerve runs in close proximity to the pudendal vessels, and intravascular injection of local anesthesia is toxic.
- If, during aspiration, blood is aspirated into the syringe, remove the needle and reinsert in a location approximately 1 cm away from the previous attempted injection site. Reattempt injection, if aspiration again occurs on the same side, abandon a third attempt even if it means the procedure for which the injection is being provided must be postponed for a day or two.
- While injection can be attempted again if attempted block fails, the toxic dose of lidocaine is 4.5 mg/kg and should not be exceeded.

11

Clitoral Hair Tourniquet Syndrome

Pauline Chang Yu and Paula J. A. Hillard

Hair tourniquet syndrome is an entity in which whereby a thread of hair wraps around an appendage causing strangulation of the appendage. It has been described involving the toe, finger, penis, and clitoris; however, clitoral or labial involvement has only been reported in 6% of all hair tourniquet cases. The average age of presentation is 5 to 9 years old. In early phases of clitoral hair tourniquet syndrome, patients may present with intermittent vulvar pain and nonspecific labia irritation. As the venous and lymphatic drainage is compromised, edema and inflammation develops. In later phases, erythematous, edematous genital mass and intense genital pain are common clinical presentations. Diagnosis can be difficult as the encircling hair may be difficult to visualize.

RELEVANT ANATOMY (Fig. 11.1)

PATIENT POSITION

- Supine on the examination table.
- "Butterfly" or "Frog-leg" position (i.e., feet placed together, knees flexed, hips abducted). In this age group, use of the stirrups or dorsal lithotomy position is typically more threatening to the child.

LANDMARKS

- Locate base of the hair tourniquet, usually embedded in the edematous tissue beneath the clitoral or labial hood.

ANESTHESIA

- Moderate sedation with narcotics and anxiolytics using pediatric protocols.
- Examination under general anesthesia may be required if exposure cannot be achieved with moderate sedation.

EQUIPMENT

- Betadine prep
- Fine-toothed forceps
- Iris scissors

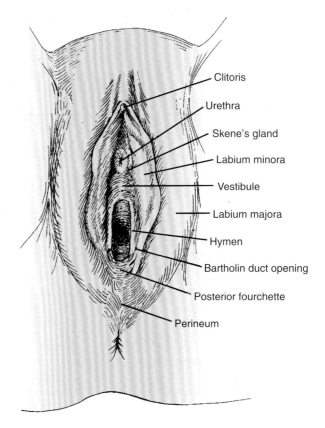

FIGURE 11.1 ● Vulva and perineum—view of external female genital anatomy showing the various structures. LifeART image copyright © 2012 Lippincott Williams & Wilkins. All rights reserved.

- Sterile 4 × 4 sponges
- Blunt probe

TECHNIQUE

1. Initiate appropriate moderate sedation for the patient with monitoring.
2. Prepare the affected area with Betadine.
3. Locate the base of the tourniquet. The strangulating hair should be visible and will be seen as a tight band of hair strangulating the clitoral base (Fig. 11.2).
4. Using the fine-toothed forceps or blunt probe, elevate or loosen the strangulating hair from the base (Fig. 11.3).
5. Use the iris scissors to cut the strangulating hair with extreme care (Fig. 11.3).
6. Alternatively, remove the hair by unwinding from the appendage.
7. Re-examine the affected area to ensure all strangulating hair is removed.

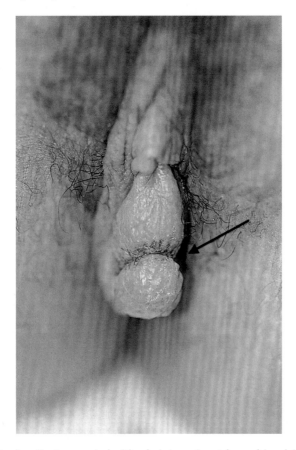

FIGURE 11.2 ● A patient presented with a hair tourniquet (*arrow*) involving the labia minora. From Fleisher GR, Ludwig S, Baskin MN. *Atlas of pediatric emergency medicine.* Philadelphia, PA: Lippincott Williams & Wilkins, 2004.

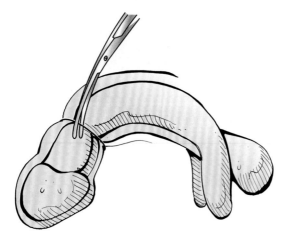

FIGURE 11.3 ● Use of iris scissors to cut the strangulating hair.

AFTERCARE

- Patient should have immediate improvement of the symptoms.
- Edema and discoloration should resolve within 30 minutes to 1 to 2 days. If reperfusion is not observed, further surgery to remove ischemic tissue may be necessary.
- Take ibuprofen and sitz bath every 6 hours as needed for pain.
- Consider a follow-up examination in 1 day, then in 1 to 2 weeks.

CPT Code

56805.   Repair of clitoris

PEARLS

- If the skin has been disrupted by the hair tourniquet, tetanus prophylaxis should be offered.
- While cases of hair tourniquets can happen spontaneously, always consider the possibility of child abuse.
- Early diagnosis and prompt treatment are essential to prevent complications such as ischemic injury, tissue necrosis, and autoamputation (Fig. 11.4).

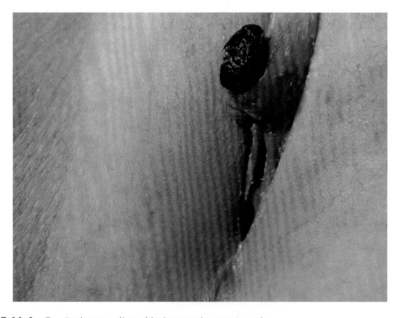

FIGURE 11.4 ● End-stage clitoral hair tourniquet necrosis.

12

Examination of the Prepubertal Female

Christine C. Picco and Paula J. A. Hillard

Examination of external genitalia is a routine portion of the physical examination for pediatricians. Internal examination is reserved for symptoms or problems of the genitourinary tract, including bleeding, itching, or discharge; speculum examination should not be performed in the office for a prepubertal child.

RELEVANT ANATOMY (Fig. 12.1)

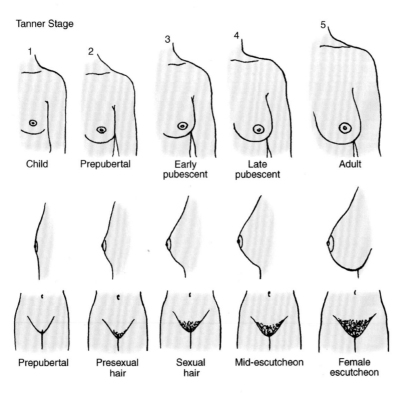

Tanner Stage

| 1 | 2 | 3 | 4 | 5 |

Child | Prepubertal | Early pubescent | Late pubescent | Adult

Prepubertal | Presexual hair | Sexual hair | Mid-escutcheon | Female escutcheon

FIGURE 12.1 ● Tanner stages in female. Rating 1 to 5. MediClip image copyright © 2012 Lippincott Williams & Wilkins. All rights reserved.

PATIENT POSITION

- Frog-leg position is optimal to evaluate vulva, on examination table or on mother's lap.
- Knee-chest position to evaluate vagina, although this may be more threatening to a child.

Landmarks (Figs. 12.2–12.4)

ANESTHESIA

- Examination under anesthesia (EUA) is necessary
  - to evaluate trauma in which the extent of a laceration cannot be visualized;
  - for unexplained bleeding;
  - if a speculum examination is required.
- Conscious sedation with monitoring can sometimes allow removal of a vaginal foreign body.

EQUIPMENT

- Otoscope may be used for external evaluation.
- Colposcope may be necessary for examination of the vulva.
- Killian nasal speculum and fiberoptic scope or hysteroscopy may be used for EUA.

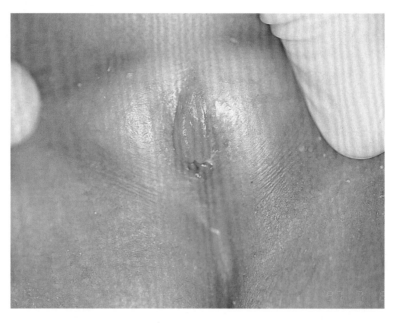

FIGURE 12.2 ● Labial adhesions. Used with permission from Fleisher GR, Ludwig S, Baskin MN, eds. *Atlas of pediatric emergency medicine.* Philadelphia, PA: Lippincott Williams & Wilkins; 2004:146.

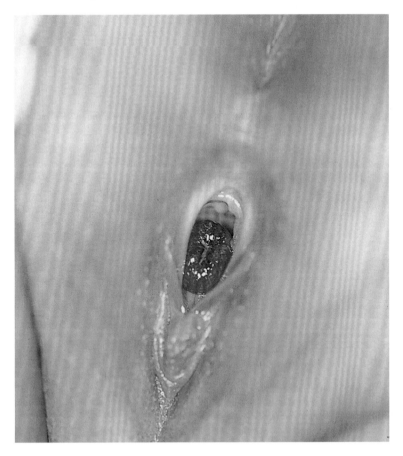

FIGURE 12.3 ● This young girl developed urethral prolapse, manifesting with the characteristic donut sign. From Fleisher GR, Ludwig S, Baskin MN. *Atlas of pediatric emergency medicine.* Philadelphia, PA: Lippincott Williams & Wilkins, 2004.

TECHNIQUE

1. Inspect external genitalia for configuration of hymen, appropriate hygiene, signs of pubertal development, rash or other lesions (condyloma, molluscum contagiosum, lichen sclerosus, labial adhesions, urethral prolapse, hair tourniquet), bleeding, or trauma (Figs. 12.2–12.4).
2. The uterus can be evaluated using a pinkie finger within the rectum and an abdominal hand.
3. Palpate inguinal areas for hernia or gonad.

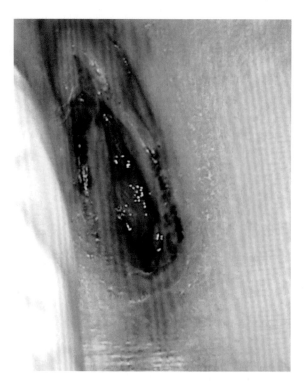

FIGURE 12.4 ● Lichen sclerosus et atrophicus. Characteristic subepidermal hemorrhages in a 4-year old with a 3-week history of genital itching and intermittent dysuria. Lesions showed only slight improvement at follow-up weeks later. Courtesy of Allan R. De Jong, MD.

AFTERCARE

1. If the examination resulted in any minor trauma to the labia, the mother should be informed, and 2% lidocaine can be used topically.

CPT Code: 99170—Anogenital examination with colposcopic magnification in childhood for suspected trauma (Note: If sexual abuse is suspected, this should only be performed by clinicians with significant experience in child sexual abuse).

PEARLS

- Speculum examination should not be performed in the office, and is generally performed with an EUA in conjunction with hysteroscopy and reserved for assessment of unexplained bleeding, trauma, or foreign body.
- Always explain to the child what they will feel with an examination.
- EUA may be needed.
- Appropriate lighting, assistance (a nurse may be required to hold an infant or toddler's legs), and explanations to the mother about how the examination differs from that of an adult will facilitate examinations.
- 2% lidocaine jelly can be used topically to allow assessment of the hymen and vaginal vestibule.

Cytology

Katherine Fuh and Paul D. Blumenthal

Worldwide, but especially in developed countries, cervical cytology remains the mainstay of cervical screening as part of cervical cancer prevention programs. Cytology is used for routine or follow-up screening for cervical cancer/precancer.

RELEVANT ANATOMY

Cervix, squamocolumnar junction. Cytologic interpretation required (Fig. 13.1.1).

PATIENT POSITION

• Dorsal lithotomy

ANESTHESIA

• None

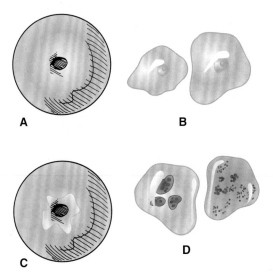

FIGURE 13.1.1 ● Papanicolaou smear. **A:** Normal appearing cervix, **B:** Normal appearing cells, **C:** Acetowhite white epithelium (possible dysplasia), **D:** Abnormal appearing (pre-cancer or cancer) cells.

EQUIPMENT (Fig. 13.1.2)

- Speculum
- Extended tip spatula/or cervical broom plus cytobrush
- Ethyl ether plus 95% ethyl alcohol or 95% ethyl alcohol alone or spray fixative (conventional)
- Slide
- Large cotton swab

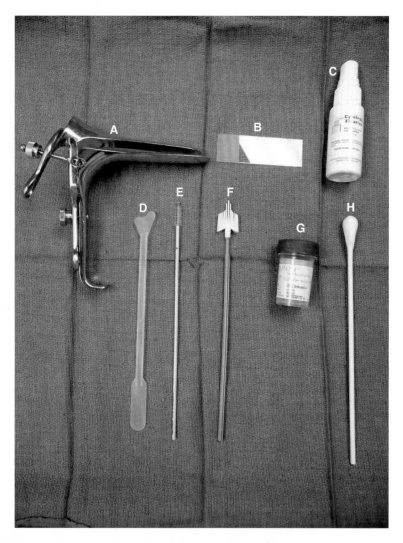

FIGURE 13.1.2 ● Cervical cytology tray. **A:** Graves or Pederson speculum, **B:** Glass slide (conventional), **C:** Fixative (conventional), **D:** Cell collection device/spatula, **E:** Cytobrush, **F:** Cell collection device ("broom"), **G:** Cell transport medium (liquid-based cytology), **H:** Procto swab.

TECHNIQUE

Conventional Cytology

1. Insert speculum—for patient comfort, small amounts of lubrication can be applied to the speculum. Large amounts of lubrication can affect quality of specimen.
2. Small amounts of blood will not interfere with cytologic sampling.
3. If performing a culture, obtain the cytology specimen first.
4. Clear the cervix of excess vaginal discharge.
5. Scrape the cervix circumferentially using a spatula (Figs. 13.1.3 and 13.1.4A).
6. Use the endocervical brush to collect the highest yield of endocervical cells (Fig. 13.1.4B).
7. Insert the brush into the endocervix so the bristles closest to the examiner are flush with the external cervical os.
8. Rotate the brush 180 degrees to obtain a sample.
9. Specimen should be rolled (brush) or smeared (spatula) uniformly onto a slide and rapidly fixed with either ethyl alcohol or spray fixative (Fig. 13.1.3C,D).

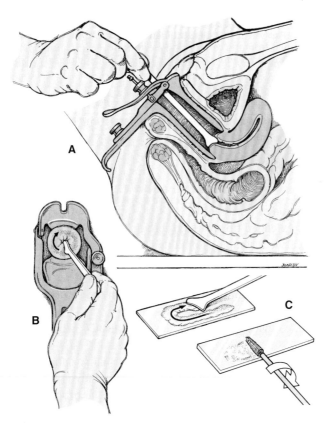

FIGURE 13.1.3 ● Pap smear. **A:** Speculum in place and Ayre spatula in position at cervical os. **B:** Tip of spatula placed in the cervical os and rotated 360 degrees. **C:** Cellular material clinging to spatula is then smeared smoothly on the glass slide, which is promptly placed in a fixative solution. **D:** Cytobrush is rotated in cervical os and rolled onto glass slide. From Neil O. Hardy, Westport, CT. From Smetlzer SC & Bare BG. *Brunner & Suddarth's textbook of medical surgical-nursing,* 8th ed Philadelphia, PA: JB Lippincott Company, 1996. Figs. 44–45.

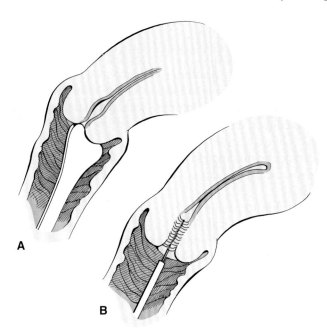

FIGURE 13.1.4 ● Pap smear. **A:** Cells obtained from transformation zone using an Ayers spatula. **B:** Cells obtained from the cervix using a cytobrush. From Gibbs RS, Karlan BY, Haney AF, et al., eds. *Danforth's obstetrics and gynecology,* 10th ed. Philadelphia, PA: Lippincott Williams & Wilkins, 2008.

10. If using a spray fixative, hold the slide at least 10 inches to prevent disruption of the cells by propellant.

Liquid-based Cytology

ThinPrep

1. Speculum insertion as noted above.
2. Either a plastic extended tip spatula or broom-like device can be used.
3. After the ectocervical sample is obtained, spatula is swirled vigorously in the vial ten times and then discarded.
4. Endocervical specimen can then be collected by inserting the endocervical brush into the canal until the bottom-most fibers touch the ectocervix. It is then rotated five times in one direction to obtain the sample.
5. If the broom-like device is used, this device is pushed gently into the endocervical canal.
6. Rotate the broom five times in one direction to obtain a sample.
7. Place the broom at the bottom of the vial of preservative solution to force the bristles to spread apart and release the sample. Swirl the broom vigorously to further release material into the vial (Fig. 13.1.5).

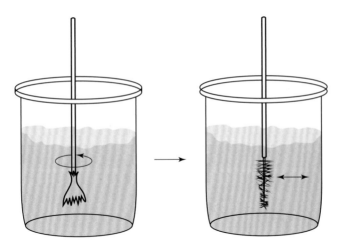

FIGURE 13.1.5 ● Pap smear. Placement of specimens in liquid collection medium. Modified from Beckmann CR, Ling FW, Smith RP, et al., eds. *Obstetrics and gynecology,* 5th ed. Philadelphia, PA: Lippincott Williams & Wilkins, 2006.

SurePath

1. Uses a special broom-type sampling device that is placed into the vial and preservative solution.
2. Insert the broom collection device into the endocervical canal using a twisting motion while applying gentle pressure and rotate five times in one direction.
3. Transfer entire sample by placing the thumb against the back of the brush pad. This will disconnect the brush from the stem.

CPT Codes: n/a

PEARLS

• With liquid-based cervical cytology co-testing for HPV and other sexually transmitted diseases using the same collection vial is possible.

Cervical Punch Biopsy

Katherine Fuh and Paul D. Blumenthal

RELEVANT ANATOMY

Cervix, squamocolumnar junction, transformation zone, acetowhite epithelium (see Figures 13.2.2, 13.2.3 and 8.1).

PATIENT POSITION

- Dorsal lithotomy

ANESTHESIA

- None

EQUIPMENT (Fig. 13.2.1)

- Speculum
- Colposcope
- 3% to 5% acetic acid
- Large cotton swabs and cotton-tip swabs
- 1% lidocaine
- 5-mL syringe
- 25-gauge 1-1/2 inch needle
- Alcohol pads
- Sterile gauze pads
- Sterile adhesive bandage
- Punch biopsy forceps (Tischler, Kevorkian, or similar)
- Formalin-filled container
- Silver nitrate or Monsel's solution

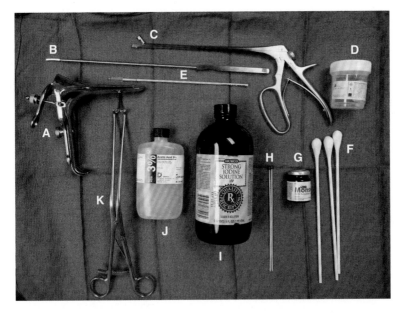

FIGURE 13.2.1 ● **A:** Graves or Pederson speculum, **B:** Endocervical curette, **C:** Tischler punch biopsy forceps, **D:** Fixative for histology (formalin), **E:** Cytobrush, **F:** Proto swabs/"pom-pom" vaginal swabs, **G:** Monsel's solution (ferrous subsulfate), **H:** Silver nitrate sticks, **I:** Lugol's iodine solution, **J:** 3% acetic acid, **K:** Cervical speculum.

TECHNIQUE (see also Colposcopy)

1. Insert speculum.
2. Cervix can be cleansed with saline-soaked cotton balls.
3. View cervix with bright light first to look for areas of erosion, true leukoplakia, pigmented lesions, areas of obvious ulceration, or exophytic growth.
4. Apply acetic acid to the cervix to enhance the definition of the squamocolumnar junction.
5. After 60 seconds, the acidic solution dehydrates cells, so squamous cells with relatively large or dense nuclei reflect light and appear white (Fig. 13.2.2A).
6. Identify the transformation zone (TZ) or squamocolumnar junction (Fig. 8.1).
7. Areas of white epithelium are further evaluated for abnormal vascular patterns such as punctation, mosaicism, or abnormal appearing vessels.
8. If no lesions are seen, a dilute Lugol's or Schiller's solution can be applied to the cervix. Uniform uptake would confirm no lesions are present. Mature, normal glycogen-containing cells will take up iodine and become dark brown. Nonglycogenated cells such as normal columnar cells or glandular cells, high grade lesions, and many low grade lesions will not take up iodine and remain yellow or "saffron" colored (Fig. 13.2.2B).
9. Use forceps to biopsy acetowhite areas and yellow-colored lesions (Fig. 13.2.3).
10. Apply silver nitrate or Monsel's solution for hemostasis.

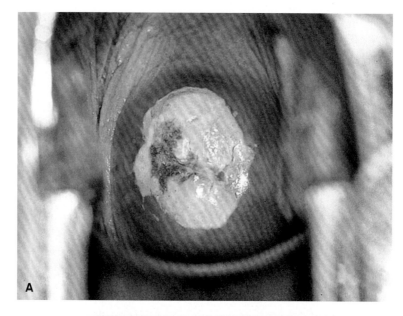

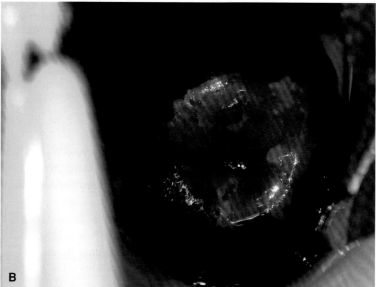

FIGURE 13.2.2 ● **A:** Acetowhite lesion after washing with acetic acid. **B:** Iodine staining revealing saffron-colored abnormal area.

AFTERCARE

- Sexual intercourse should be avoided for several days after the biopsy to minimize trauma to the cervix and possible infection.

CPT Code

57500. Biopsy of cervix, single or multiple, or local excision of lesion, with or without fulguration (separate procedure)

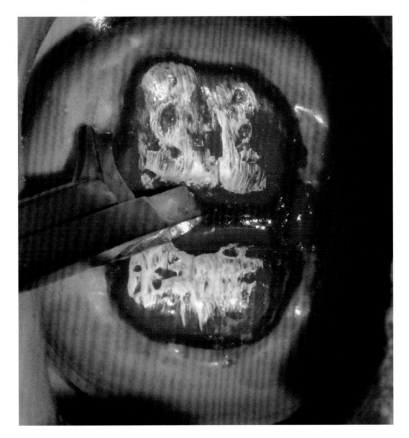

FIGURE 13.2.3 ● Biopsy forceps applied to acetowhite lesion on cervix.

PEARLS

• Efficacy of colposcopy depends upon the experience and training of the colposcopist.
• Columnar cells and blood vessels are not affected by acetic acid.
• The transformation zone represents the area of active cell division and therefore the region that is most likely to display abnormal growth.
• Green filter light examination accentuates abnormal vasculature by darkening blood vessels and sharpens the contrast between vessels and surrounding epithelium.
• Cervical biopsies should be taken from inferior to superior to avoid having bleeding from biopsy sites obscure subsequent biopsies.
• Each specimen is labeled individually according to its location on the cervix like the face of a clock.
• Biopsies are relatively contraindicated in patients on anticoagulants, have a known bleeding disorder, or who are pregnant. If a biopsy is necessary, appropriate steps should be taken to minimize bleeding and to treat heavy bleeding.
• Monsel's solution and silver nitrate can interfere with interpretation of the biopsy specimen, so these should not be applied until all biopsies have been taken.

13.3

Cryosurgery/Cryotherapy

Katherine Fuh and Paul D. Blumenthal

RELEVANT ANATOMY

Cervix, transformation zone, squamocolumnar junction, internal cervical os, limits of cervical lesion.

PATIENT POSITION

- Dorsal lithotomy

ANESTHESIA

- None

EQUIPMENT

- Speculum
- 5% acetic acid
- Cervical probe (shallow, convex probe [5 mm depth] preferable)
- Cryosurgery unit (cryounit, cryotip, refrigerant)

TECHNIQUE

1. Ensure that adequate refrigerant (nitrous oxide or carbon dioxide) is present in the tank (Fig. 13.3.1).
2. Place speculum.
3. Visualize entire exocervix.
4. Confirm colposcopic assessment (repeat if necessary).
5. If the lesion is more than 1½ times the surface area of the probe tip, or the probe tip will not completely cover the lesion, the lesion should be subdivided and each segment individually frozen.
6. Apply cryoprobe to cervix. Put moderate pressure on cervix to get firm contact (Figs. 13.3.2A,B).
7. Turn on refrigerant flow. An ice ball should start forming over the next 30 seconds (Fig. 13.3.3).
8. Single freeze technique: One application of the cryoprobe for 5 minutes.
9. Double freeze technique: Two applications of 3 minutes each with a 5-minute intermission between applications.

76

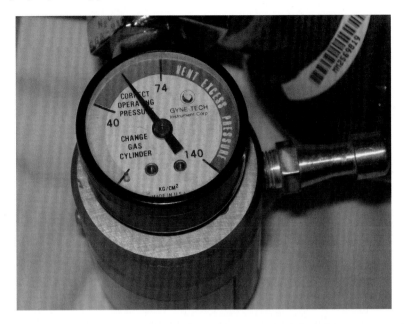

FIGURE 13.3.1 ● Gauge showing adequate refrigerant in tank (needle in green area).

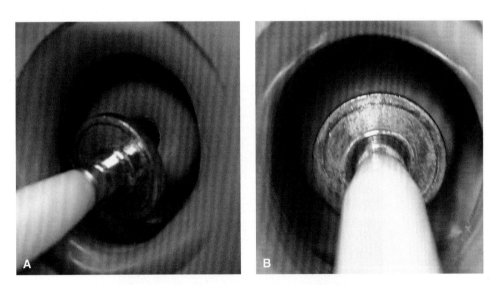

FIGURE 13.3.2 ● **A:** Cryoprobe being placed onto cervix. **B:** Cryoprobe centered on cervix and pressure applied.

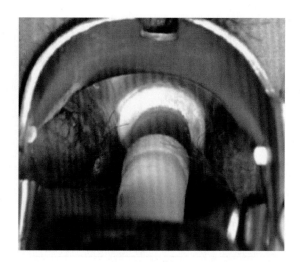

FIGURE 13.3.3 ● "Iceball" forming on cervix as refrigerant is applied.

10. Confirmation of an adequate ice ball can be made by "percussing" the ice ball with the wooden end of a Q-tip (Fig. 13.3.4).
11. Once entire area of abnormal tissue has been clearly frozen, engage the defrost mechanism of the cryounit and once defrosting has occurred, disengage the probe.
12. Speculum is removed.

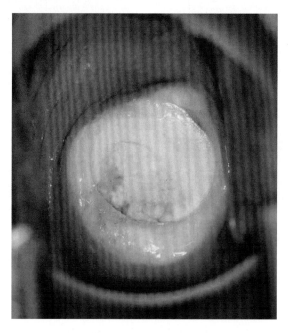

FIGURE 13.3.4 ● Satisfactory "iceball" on cervix at end procedure.

AFTERCARE

- Watery vaginal discharge generally continues for several weeks after treatment.
- If patients find the discharge bothersome, the necrotic tissue can be removed from the cervix using ring forceps.

CPT Code

57511.   Cautery of cervix; cryocautery, initial or repeat

PEARLS

- Actual duration of the freezing is not necessarily timed and the times listed above are guidelines.
- It is more important to make certain that the edge of the ice ball extends at least 5 to 6 mm past the edge of the probe onto normal-appearing epithelium.
- The cryotip must *not* come in contact with the vaginal vault. If necessary use tongue depressors or cytology spatulas to separate the vagina from the lateral vaginal walls. Use wooden devices since they will not conduct the cold, nor will they crack.

Loop Electrosurgical Excision Procedure (LEEP)

Katherine Fuh and Paul D. Blumenthal

RELEVANT ANATOMY

Cervix, transformation zone, squamocolumnar junction, internal cervical os, limits of cervical lesion.

PATIENT POSITION

- Dorsal lithotomy

ANESTHESIA

- Paracervical block—1% lidocaine (Refer to Chapter 13.7 and Figures 13.7.1 and 13.7.2)

EQUIPMENT

- Loop electrode–size dependent on area to excise
- Electrosurgical generator
- Grounding pad
- Nonconductive Graves speculum with integrated smoke tube
- Suction tubing
- 5% acetic acid
- Lugol's solution
- Long cotton swabs
- Endocervical curette
- Ball electrode
- Monsel's paste/solution
- Tissue forceps
- Formalin container
- Suture
- Needle driver
- Scissors
- Supplies for paracervical block

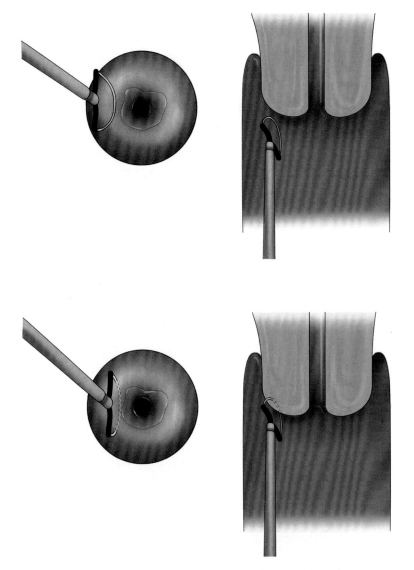

FIGURE 13.4.1 ● Loop electrode being positioned over area to be excised (**top**) and initial insertion of probe into cervical tissue (**bottom**). From Mayeaux EJ, Jr. Loop electrosurgical excisional procedure. In: Mayeaux EJ, Jr, ed. *The essential guide to primary care procedures.* Philadelphia, PA: Lippincott Williams & Wilkins, 2009:607–617.

TECHNIQUE

1. Place grounding pad horizontally over patient's thigh.
2. Place speculum with suction tubing connected. Cleanse cervix and perform paracervical block.
3. Place acetic acid on the cervix.
4. Excise area of acetowhite lesion. Alternatively, Lugol's solution may be applied to identify and excise lesion.
5. Set electrosurgical generator at 30 to 40 W on "blend 1." (Other settings may be used such as 80 W "pure cut.")

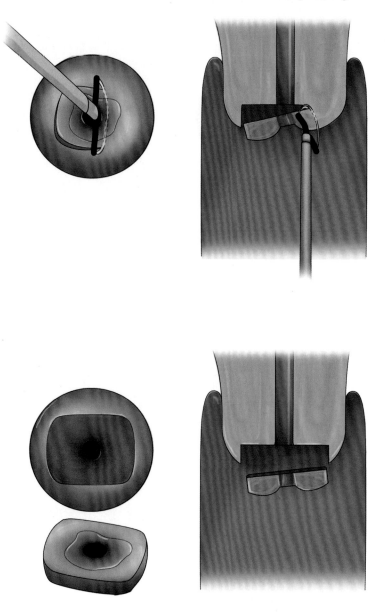

FIGURE 13.4.2 ● Loop electrode being passed through cervical stroma under the transformation zone (**top**) resulting in an excisional biopsy (**bottom**). From Mayeaux EJ, Jr. Loop electrosurgical excisional procedure. In: Mayeaux EJ, Jr, ed. *The essential guide to primary care procedures.* Philadelphia, PA: Lippincott Williams & Wilkins, 2009:607–617.

6. Place normal saline on the exocervix to rehydrate the tissue and decrease risk of
   loop electrode sticking to tissue.
7. Loop is carefully passed simultaneously around and under the transformation zone,
   thus excising it. The loop should be allowed to glide through the cervix from one side
   to the other, allowing the cutting current to divide the tissue (Figs. 13.4.1–13.4.3).

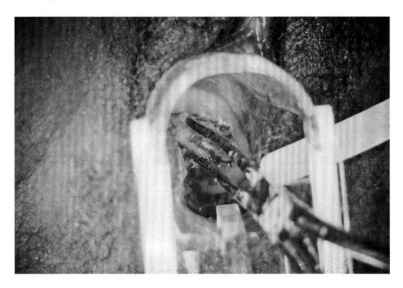

FIGURE 13.4.3 ● Forceps being used to remove excised tissue. From Mayeaux EJ, Jr. Loop electrosurgical excisional procedure. In: Mayeaux EJ, Jr, ed. *The essential guide to primary care procedures.* Philadelphia, PA: Lippincott Williams & Wilkins, 2009:607–617.

8. If the lesion extends into the endocervical canal beyond the reach of the loop, additional tissue may be excised with a smaller-diameter rectangular loop ("high hat") (Fig. 13.4.4).
9. Remove the specimen in the correct orientation.
10. Place a suture at 12 o'clock on the excised specimen to orient for histopathologic analysis.
11. Achieve hemostasis at the base of the specimen with coagulation using the 5-mm ball electrode and Monsel's paste/solution.

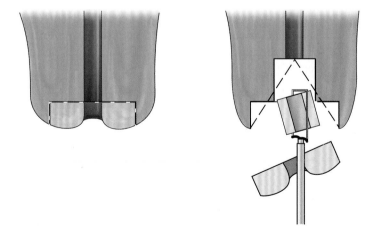

FIGURE 13.4.4 ● Rectangular probe being used to excise tissue from higher in the endo-cervical canal. From Mayeaux EJ, Jr. Loop electrosurgical excisional procedure. In: Mayeaux EJ, Jr, ed. *The essential guide to primary care procedures.* Philadelphia, PA: Lippincott Williams & Wilkins, 2009:607–617.

AFTERCARE

- The patient is instructed to avoid intercourse and place nothing in the vagina, and not immerse herself in water (e.g., take a bath or swim) for 2 to 4 weeks. She is seen in the office at 6 weeks.
- If Monsel's solution was used, remind the patient that she will have brown, grainy-like discharge for several days.

CPT Code

57522. Conization of cervix, with or without fulguration, with or without dilation and curettage, with or without repair; loop electrode excision

PEARLS

- A blended current mixes cutting and coagulating currents.
- The higher the blend, the more the coagulating current and the greater the thermal damage.
- If the surgeon attempts to pull too quickly through the cervix, the loop will drag, bend, or adhere to the tissue, resulting in a shallower excision than was intended. If the loop moves too slowly, however, excess thermal damage to the specimen will occur. Application of saline onto the exocervix further decreases this risk.
- If hemostasis is difficult to achieve with the ball electrode and Monsel's paste, sutures may be necessary.
  - Place a suture at 3 o'clock and 9 o'clock. This must be performed at a distal point on the cervix to avoid ureteral compromise and may reduce bleeding by reducing pulse pressure from the cervical artery. Place Gelfoam at the base and tie the suture across the front of the cervix to keep the Gelfoam in place.
- Follow-up in 6 weeks to assess cervical healing, but no action should be taken with respect to dysplasia at this time.
- If colposcopy was satisfactory, an assessment of cervical cytology with or without colposcopy is performed approximately 6 months postoperatively. This should not be performed before 4 months since any specimens obtained at this time are frequently contaminated with debris, metaplastic cells, and leukocytes. If either colposcopy was unsatisfactory or LEEP (Loop Electrosurgical Excision Procedure) was performed for a recurrent CIN II/III lesion, HPV testing is performed at 6 and 12 months postoperatively.

Laser Ablation

Katherine Fuh and Paul D. Blumenthal

Histologically proven precancerous lesion(s) on the cervix, are candidates for laser ablation. Given the efficacy and availability of LEEP for diagnostic purposes Laser conization procedures are no longer a preferred approach to diagnostic excisional biopsy.

RELEVANT ANATOMY

Cervix, transformation zone, squamocolumnar junction, internal cervical os, limits of cervical lesion.

PATIENT POSITION

- Dorsal lithotomy

ANESTHESIA

- Paracervical block

EQUIPMENT

- CO_2 laser
- Operating microscope used to direct the beam to target tissue
- Vacuum device
- Nonreflective, coated speculum
- 5% acetic acid

TECHNIQUE

1. Place anti-reflective, coated speculum into the vagina and orient for optimum cervical exposure.
2. Turn on vacuum for smoke/vapor removal.
3. Place 5% acetic acid on the cervix and note limits of lesion, correlating with previous colposcopic impressions as needed.
4. Vaporize acetowhite lesions or the entire transformation zone using continuous beam and settings of 10 W with a spot size of 1 mm.
5. Ensure that: (1) Upper limits (in canal) have been vaporized and (2) adequate hemostasis.

AFTERCARE

- The patient is instructed to avoid intercourse and place nothing in the vagina, and not immerse herself in water (e.g., take a bath or swim) for 2 to 4 weeks. She is seen in the office at 6 weeks.
- If Monsel's solution was used, remind the patient that she may have brown grainy discharge for several days.

CPT Code
57513.   Cautery of cervix; laser ablation

PEARLS

- Laser is an acronym for Light Amplification by Stimulated Emission of Radiation.
- CO_2 laser produces electromagnetic radiation by a high density, controlled discharge of a mixture of carbon dioxide, nitrogen, and helium gas.
- This energy is emitted at a wavelength of 10.6 μ with an average power of 10 to 10,000 W. Vaporization of biologic tissue is achieved with little difficulty.
- Tissue destruction is achieved by raising the temperature of the cell until intracellular water turns to steam, vaporizing the cell.
- Entire transformation zone must be destroyed in order to have improved treatment success.
- Some discomfort after laser therapy is common, but healing is rapid and scarring minimal.
- Standard methods for hemostasis such as silver nitrate or Monsel's solution application can be used as needed (see also LEEP).

Dilation for Cervical Stenosis

Katherine Fuh and Paul D. Blumenthal

Cervical dilation may be required when visualization of the endocervix is impaired by apparent or functional stenosis or migration of the squamocolumnar junction (SCJ) into the canal or when access to the endometrial cavity is required as for endometrial biopsy, abortion, or intrauterine contraceptive device (IUD) insertion.

RELEVANT ANATOMY

Cervix, external cervical os, internal cervical os.

PATIENT POSITION

- Dorsal lithotomy

ANESTHESIA

- None

EQUIPMENT

- Misoprostol 200 mcg buccally 2 hours before if planned ahead
- Pratt dilators (preferred) or Hegar dilators (Fig. 13.6.1)
- Lacrimal duct probes or "os finder" for complicated cases of stenosis
- Single tooth tenaculum or atraumatic vulsellum forceps
- Lubrication
- Speculum
- Equipment/instruments for paracervical block

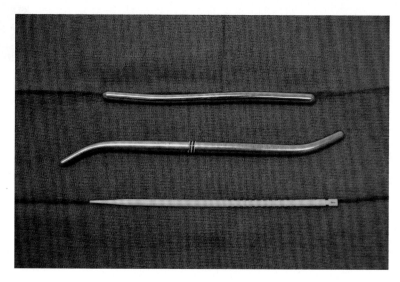

FIGURE 13.6.1 ● Dilators for dilating cervical canal. Dilators are generally inserted to a point just beyond the cervical isthmus (internal os). **Top:** Hegar Dilator. **Middle:** Pratt dilator. **Bottom:** "os finder".

TECHNIQUE

1. A paracervical block may be placed prior to cervical dilation procedures in order to reduce procedural discomfort (see Chapter 13.7, Paracervical Block).
2. Place a single tooth tenaculum on the anterior or posterior portion of the cervix.
3. Grasp the dilator in the middle with the thumb and index finger.
4. Dilator should be inserted just through the internal os without entering the uterine cavity more deeply than necessary.
5. Place lubrication at the tip of the dilator.
6. Start with a 13F Pratt dilator or a 1-mm Hegar dilator.

CPT Code

57800. Dilation of cervical canal, instrumental (separate procedure)

PEARLS

- Pratt dilator sizes range from 13 to 43F; each French unit is equivalent to 0.33 mm in diameter. It is characterized by a gradual taper at the end of the instrument.
- Hegar dilators have a blunt end and have sizes ranging from 1 to 26 mm in diameter.
- Pratt dilators have been shown to require less force for dilation and are less likely to cause a perforation of the uterus.
- An "os finder" (a tapered, flexible plastic device) can be used when just finding the os is necessary. Its flexible and tapered nature can reduce trauma and provide enhanced "feel" for the location of the internal os.

Paracervical Block

Katherine Fuh and Paul D. Blumenthal

RELEVANT ANATOMY

Exocervix, posterior cul de sac, uterosacral ligaments.

PATIENT POSITION

- Dorsal lithotomy

EQUIPMENT

- Single tooth tenaculum or atraumatic vulsellum forceps
- 1% lidocaine maximum volume of 20 mL
- 10-cc syringe
- 22 to 23G need on extender or spinal needle
- Speculum

TECHNIQUE

1. Place speculum to obtain good visualization of the entire cervix.
2. Place 2 to 3 mL of lidocaine at the 6 or 12 o'clock position (depending on where tenaculum placement is planned).
3. Grasp the anesthetized portion of the cervix with a tenaculum or atraumatic vulsellum forceps.
4. Inject 10 cc of lidocaine at or just above each uterosacral ligament (4 o'clock and 8 o'clock position) 1 cm under the mucosa where vagina reflects off the cervix (Figs. 13.7.1 and 13.7.2).
5. Inspect the injection sites for bleeding.
6. May need to hold pressure with a long cotton swab or silver nitrate.
7. Wait 10 minutes before proceeding with the procedure.

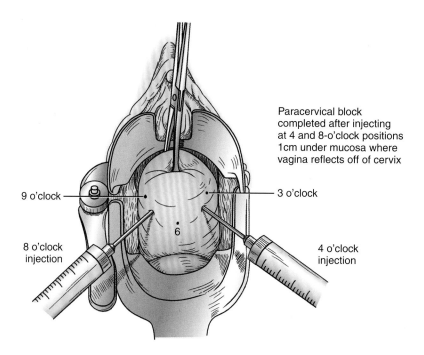

Paracervical block completed after injecting at 4 and 8-o'clock positions 1cm under mucosa where vagina reflects off of cervix

9 o'clock — • • — 3 o'clock

• 6

8 o'clock injection

4 o'clock injection

FIGURE 13.7.1 ● Relevant anatomy for paracervical block. From Shulman LP, Ling FW. Surgical termination of pregnancy. In: Mann WJ, Stovall TG, eds. *Gynecologic surgery.* Churchill Livingstone, Inc, 1996:799.

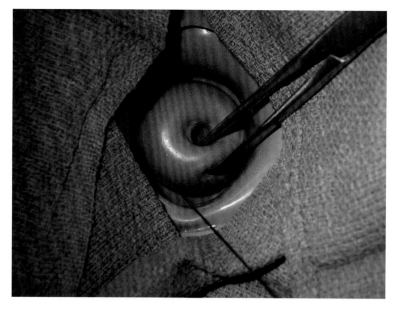

FIGURE 13.7.2 ● Needle being inserted at the 8 o'clock position just above the uterosacral ligament.

CPT Code

64435.   Injection, anesthetic agent; paracervical (uterine) nerve

PEARLS

- Maximum dose of lidocaine is 4.5 mg/kg body weight.
- Peak plasma level occurs in 10 to 15 minutes.
- Epinephrine 1:200,000 or 5 mcg/mL added to local anesthetics can cause vasoconstriction. As a result, there is decreased bleeding at the operative site, an increase in the potency of the block, and prolongation of duration of the anesthesia.
- Risks of systemic epinephrine administration can cause cardiostimulatory effects particularly in patients who are hypertensive or prone to cardiac tachyarrhythmias.
- Grasping the cervix on the posterior lip allows for better access to the portions of the cervix where the local is to be injected (4 and 8 o'clock) and obviates the need to keep lifting the tenaculum out of the way during the subsequent procedure. Posterior lip placement has no adverse effect on accessing the cervical canal or the uterus of an anteverted or anteflexed uterus.

Endometrial Biopsy

Thuong-Thuong Nguyen and Paul D. Blumenthal

Office-based endometrial sampling with devices such as the Pipelle Endometrial Aspirator®, Explora Curette, Vabra Aspirator®, Endo Sampler®, and Novak Curette, is a safer, more convenient, less expensive, and reliable alternative to dilation and curettage.

RELEVANT ANATOMY

Same as for IUD insertion

PATIENT POSITION

- Dorsal lithotomy

LANDMARKS

- Cervix and cervical os

ANESTHESIA

- Paracervical block can provide some relief from this brief procedure but is rarely necessary.
- Ibuprofen.
- Laminaria/misoprostol can be helpful in cases of cervical stenosis.

EQUIPMENT

- Speculum
- Tenaculum or atraumatic vulsellum forceps
- Uterine sound
- Lacrimal duct dilators or 1- to-4 mm cervical dilators
- Betadine solution or swabs
- Large cotton swabs or ring forceps and clean gauze
- Formalin solution for pathology
- Endometrial biopsy device (Fig. 14.1)
  - Pipelle de Cornier Endometrial Aspirator: A disposable and flexible polypropylene endometrial suction curette that is 3 mm in diameter with a distal side port to

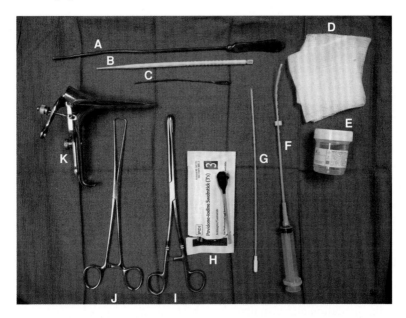

FIGURE 14.1 ● Endometrial sample biopsy tray. **A:** uterine sound, **B:** cervical os finder; **C:** filiform dilator, **D:** 4 × 4 sponge, **E:** formalin solution, **F:** endosampler device with locking plunger and 5 cc syringe, **G:** Pipelle endometrial sampler, **H:** povidone iodine swabs, **I:** ring forceps, **J:** single-toothed tenaculum, **K:** Graves or Pederson speculum.

collect tissue. Withdrawal of the piston from the sheath creates suction. Advantages: Easy to use and generally well tolerated by patients. Disadvantage: Smaller sample size compared to D& C.

- Explora Curette: A 3-mm disposable plastic device that is attached to a syringe. Once the curette is advanced to the uterine fundus, a syringe is attached to the cannula. The plunger of the syringe is pulled back and locked to create negative pressure. The curette has an outer diameter of 3.0 mm and is slightly more rigid than the Pipelle device. This cannula has a sharp Randall-type cutting edge on the distal end, on one side of the cannula. Advantages: Rigidity of catheter enables operator to negotiate a stenotic cervical os and larger sample size compared to Pipelle. Disadvantage: Smaller sample size compared to D& C.
- Vabra Aspirator: A 4-mm disposable plastic or a 2- to 3-mm stainless device is attached to an external vacuum pump. The tissue is removed from a trap, and then placed in formalin. Procedure is otherwise similar to that of the Pipelle. Advantages: Larger tissue samples obtained than with Pipelle, similar to D& C. Disadvantages: More uncomfortable and vacuum is noisy.
- Karman Cannula: A flexible 4- to 6-mm plastic device with two distal ports is attached to a reusable syringe or vacuum pump. Similar advantages and disadvantages to Vabra.
- Novak Curette: A 2- to 4-mm stainless steel device is attached to a plunger that creates suction when pulled back. Disadvantage: Uncomfortable.
- Silver nitrate sticks or Monsel's solution for hemostasis

TECHNIQUE

Pretreatment and Preparation

- No antibiotics are necessary.
- Recommend NSAIDs such as ibuprofen 600 to 800 mg 30 to 60 minutes prior to procedure.
- Misoprostol 200 mcg buccally the night prior to the procedure if cervical stenosis is anticipated in a premenopausal patient.
- Consider a paracervical block with 10 cc of 1% or 2% lidocaine without epinephrine to reduce uterine cramping.
- Perform a preprocedure bimanual examination to assess for uterine anteversion or retroversion. This will aid in guidance of the sampling device through the cervical canal and may decrease the risk of uterine perforation.

PROCEDURE

Pipelle

1. Place the speculum and visualize the cervix.
2. Prep the cervix with Betadine.
   a. If a tenaculum is required for positioning of the cervix or for traction, grasp the anterior or posterior lip of the cervix slowly with the teeth oriented horizontally in the conventional fashion or vertically across the cervical os. Alternatively, grasp the posterior lip of a retroverted uterus. If the cervix is parous and space permits, an atraumatic vulsellum forceps can be used.
   b. If the Pipelle does not pass easily through the os, gently dilate the cervix with a lacrimal duct dilator, 1- to-4 mm cervical dilators, or a uterine sound. Alternatively, use an Explora Curette in lieu of the Pipelle.
3. The depth of the uterus can be measured with the curette sheath, which is marked in centimeters (Fig. 14.2).
4. Insert the Pipelle with piston in place.
5. Using steady pressure, pass the Pipelle through the cervical canal, applying counter traction with the tenaculum, if needed. Stop advancing the Pipelle through the uterine cavity once there is resistance, usually indicating the fundus has been reached. Note the markings for depth on the sheath (Fig. 14.3).
6. Gently let the tenaculum handle rest. Then use one hand to steady the sheath, and the other to pull completely back on the piston to create the suction (Fig. 14.4).
7. Rotate the sheath 360 degrees while passing the distal end with the tissue sampling port back and forth between the internal os and the fundus. Attempt to make one complete pass from fundus to internal os per 90 degrees. Avoid withdrawing the sheath completely, thereby losing suction (Figs. 14.5, 14.6).
8. Remove the sheath once sufficient tissue is seen within the Pipelle.
9. Without contaminating the tip, position the Pipelle over the formalin container and expel the tissue by pushing the piston back into the sheath (Fig. 14.7).
   a. If there is insufficient tissue for diagnosis, a second pass can be made for more tissue if the tip was not contaminated.

---

*If the cervix is parous and centered in the visual field, the Pipelle can sometimes be passed without placement of a tenaculum or cervical dilation.

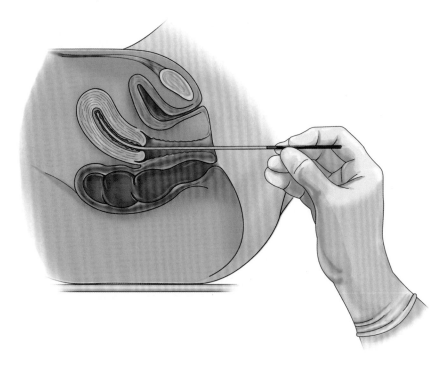

FIGURE 14.2 ● Uterus being sounded with sampling device. From Mayeaux EJ. Endometrial biopsy. In: Mayeaux EJ, ed. The Essential Guide to Primary Care Procedures. Philadelphia, PA: Lippincott Williams & Wilkins, 2009.

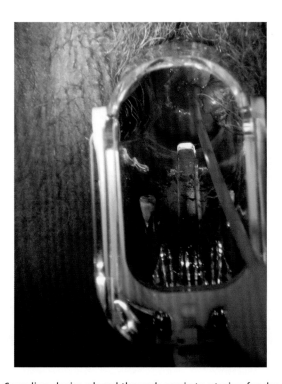

FIGURE 14.3 ● Sampling device placed through cervix to uterine fundus. From Mayeaux EJ. Endometrial biopsy. In: Mayeaux EJ, ed. The Essential Guide to Primary Care Procedures. Philadelphia, PA: Lippincott Williams & Wilkins, 2009.

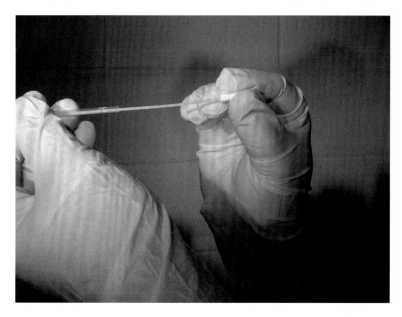

FIGURE 14.4 ● Piston of sampling device being pulled back to create vacuum. From Mayeaux EJ. Endometrial biopsy. In: Mayeaux EJ, ed. The Essential Guide to Primary Care Procedures. Philadelphia, PA: Lippincott Williams & Wilkins, 2009.

10. Gently remove the tenaculum, if one has been placed, and apply pressure to any bleeding sites with large cotton swabs or a sponge stick. An advantage of an atraumatic vulsellum forceps is that it does not pierce the cervix and therefore, at end procedure, there is no bleeding. Additional hemostasis can be obtained with silver nitrate sticks or Monsel's solution, but this is rarely necessary.

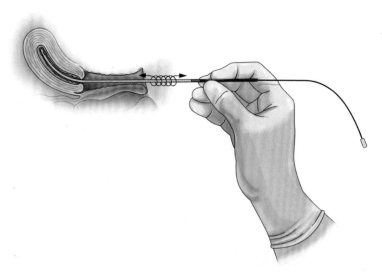

FIGURE 14.5 ● Using combination of rotating and in and out movements of the sampling device to obtain specimen. From Mayeaux EJ. Endometrial biopsy. In: Mayeaux EJ, ed. The Essential Guide to Primary Care Procedures. Philadelphia, PA: Lippincott Williams & Wilkins, 2009.

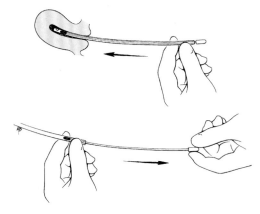

FIGURE 14.6 ● Endometrial biopsy using Pipelle. Hollow tube held in uterine cavity as stylet/piston is withdrawn generating aspiration. From Charles RB Beckmann, Frank W, et al. Obstetrics and Gynecology, 5th ed. Philadelphia, PA: Lippincott Williams & Wilkins, 2006.

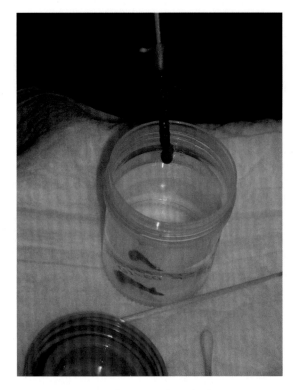

FIGURE 14.7 ● Expressing specimen from sampling device. From Mayeaux EJ. Endometrial biopsy. In: Mayeaux EJ, ed. The Essential Guide to Primary Care Procedures. Philadelphia, PA: Lippincott Williams & Wilkins, 2009.

Side Effects and Complications

- Most commonly, transient cramping. Manage with NSAIDs pre- and postprocedure. Pain should resolve in 12 hours.
- Vasovagal reaction. Reposition the patient to a more comfortable supine position and allow her to rest until she does not feel light headed. Check vital signs. Offer juice, if available.
- Bleeding. Apply pressure, silver nitrate sticks, or Monsel's solution. Advise the patient that she may expect some bleeding or spotting after the procedure.
- Rarely: Uterine perforation, severe bleeding, pelvic infection, bacteremia.

AFTERCARE

- Recommend NSAIDs for cramping pain.
- Patient should notify MD with any persistent pain for over 48 hours not relieved with medication, heavy vaginal bleeding, foul-smelling vaginal discharge, fevers, or chills.
- No restrictions on activities or intercourse.

CPT Codes

58100.   Endometrial sampling (biopsy) with or without endocervical sampling (biopsy), without cervical dilation, any method (separate procedure)

58110.   Endometrial sampling (biopsy) performed in conjunction with colposcopy (list separately in addition to code for primary procedure)

PEARLS

- Always perform a bimanual examination before starting EMB to determine if the uterus is anteverted or retroverted.
- The Pipelle can be molded gently while still within the sterile packaging to briefly conform to the direction of the uterus (i.e., anteverted, retroverted).

Office Hysteroscopy

Brooke E. Friedman and Mary T. Jacobson

Hysteroscopy is a procedure in which an imaging scope provides visualization of the vagina, cervix, endometrial cavity, and tubal ostia. With hysteroscopy, one can diagnose pathology and often treat concurrently. In the office setting, smaller-diameter hysteroscopic equipment can be used with minimal to moderate sedation and analgesia, thus avoiding the costs and inconveniences of scheduling in the operating room.

RELEVANT ANATOMY (Fig. 15.1.1)

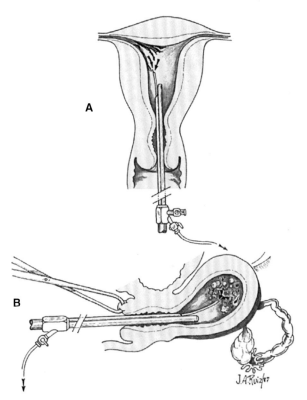

FIGURE 15.1.1 ● Correct positioning of the hysteroscope in the uterus. A polyethylene tube can be inserted through the hysteroscopic operating channel for aspiration of debris, blood clots, mucus, and air bubbles when using liquid media. **A:** Anteroposterior view. **B:** Sagittal view. From Baggish MS, Valle RF, Guedj H. *Hysteroscopy: visual perspectives of uterine anatomy, physiology, and pathology.* Philadelphia, PA: Lippincott Williams & Wilkins, 2007.

PATIENT POSITION

- The patient should lie in dorsal lithotomy position with her feet in stirrups.

LANDMARKS

- Bimanual examination is performed to determine if the uterus is anteverted or retroverted.
- The cervix must be visualized with a speculum.

ANESTHESIA

- Cervical block with 5 cc per injection site of 1% lidocaine (see Chapter 13.7, Paracervical Block).
- 1 to 2 cc of 1% lidocaine into the site of tenaculum or vulsellum forceps placement.
- If necessary, a combination of ketorolac with either hydrocodone/acetaminophen and diazepam, or IV fentanyl and midazolam may be used in conjunction with the block.

EQUIPMENT (Fig. 15.1.2A–C)

- Hysteroscope, consisting of eyepiece, barrel, and objective lens
- Light generator and fiber optic light cable
- Camera
- Diagnostic sheath (required to deliver the distending media)
- Operative sheath (optional depending on procedure)
- Distending media (e.g., CO_2 gas, electrolyte- or nonelectrolyte-containing solution)
- Distending inflow and outflow tubing or CO_2 insufflation tubing designed for hysteroscopy
- Accessory instruments (e.g., alligator grasping forceps, biopsy forceps)

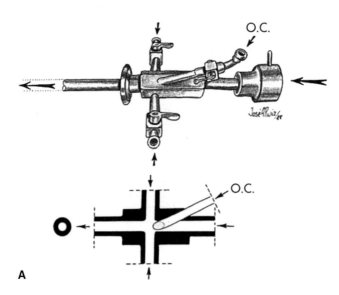

FIGURE 15.1.2 ● "Anatomy" of an hysteroscope and imaging system. **A:** An operating sheath with two stopcocks. The operating channel (O.C.) feeds into a common channel (*arrow*). A rubber nipple prevents the loss of distending medium when an operating device is inserted. From Baggish MS, Valle RF, Guedj H. *Hysteroscopy: visual perspectives of uterine anatomy, physiology and pathology.* Philadelphia: Lippincott Williams & Wilkins, 2007.

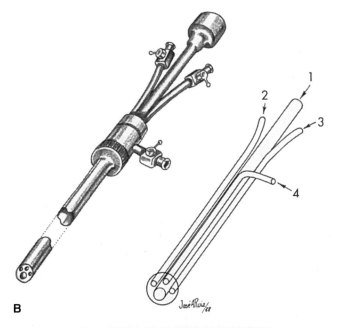

B

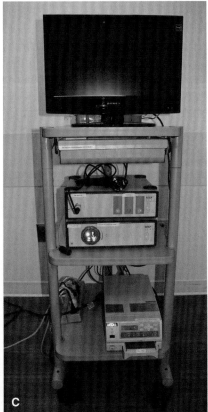

C

FIGURE 15.1.2 *(Continued)* ● **B:** Dual operating channel sheath permits aspiration and operating at the same time. The sheath consists of four isolated channels: Telescope (1); operating (2); operating (3); medium instillation (4). From Baggish MS, Valle RF, Guedj H. *Hysteroscopy: visual perspectives of uterine anatomy, physiology and pathology*. Philadelphia: Lippincott Williams & Wilkins, 2007. **C:** This endoscopic cart contains a light source, photographic equipment, and video monitor.

TECHNIQUE

1. Insert an open-sided bivalve speculum into the vagina. Alternatively, a weighted speculum and right angle retractor can be used, although this is more uncomfortable in an awake patient.
2. Cleanse the vagina and cervix with povidone–iodine, using soaked sterile sponges on a long ring forceps.
3. Inject 1 to 2 mL of lidocaine intracervically, noting the presence of a wheal on the exocervix, usually at the 6 or 12 o'clock position (wherever the tenaculum will be placed).
4. Grasp the cervix with a tenaculum, ring, or vulsellum forceps at the site where the local had just been injected.
5. Perform a two- or four-quadrant cervical block using 20 mL of 1% lidocaine at the 2 o'clock, 4 o'clock, 8 o'clock, and 10 o'clock positions.
6. Remove all instruments from the vagina and wait 10 to 15 minutes to allow the local anesthesia to take effect.
7. Reinsert the sterile speculum and repeat step 2.
8. Sequentially dilate the cervix up to the desired dilation to accommodate the hysteroscopic diameter.
9. Take care not to dilate the cervix beyond the diameter of the hysteroscope, as this may cause leakage of distending medium and suboptimal visualization of the uterine cavity.
10. Purge air from all tubing before inserting the hysteroscope and avoid Trendelenburg position, in order to minimize risk of a gas embolus.
11. While infusing media, insert the hysteroscope into the cervical canal, carefully advancing into the uterine cavity under direct visualization, watching the video monitor (Fig. 15.1.3).
12. Remove the speculum in order to facilitate movement of the hysteroscope.

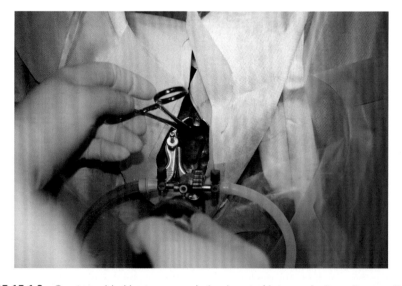

FIGURE 15.1.3 ● Assembled hysteroscope being inserted into cervix. From Berman JM, Shavell VI. Office hysteroscopy. In: Mayeaux EJ, ed. *The essential guide to primary care procedures.* Philadelphia, PA: Lippincott Williams & Wilkins, 2009.

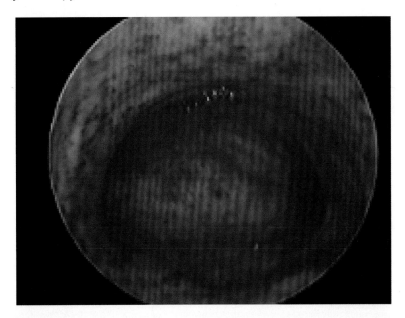

FIGURE 15.1.4 ● Initial view of uterine cavity and anterior wall. From Berman JM, Shavell VI. Office hysteroscopy. In: Mayeaux EJ, ed. *The essential guide to primary care procedures.* Philadelphia, PA: Lippincott Williams & Wilkins, 2009.

13. Perform a systematic inspection, noting the bilateral tubal ostia, uterine cavity contour, endometrium, and any pathology (Figs. 15.1.4–15.1.7).
14. Rotate the hysteroscope on its long axis (i.e., by rotating the light post) to obtain complete visualization of the uterine cavity instead of torquing the hysteroscope to minimize patient discomfort. It is helpful to document findings with photographs.
15. If applicable, perform the intended operative hysteroscopic procedure.
16. Be mindful of the hysteroscopic fluid deficit. The fluid deficit thresholds are as follows.
    - Electrolyte solution: 750 mL: Plan completion of procedure; 2,500 mL: Stop procedure (or earlier in patients who are elderly or have comorbidities).
    - Nonelectrolyte: 750 mL: Plan completion of procedure or stop procedure in patients who are elderly or have comorbidities; 1,500 mL: Stop procedure.
17. Remove all instruments from the vagina.

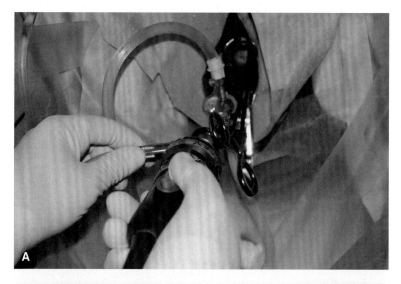

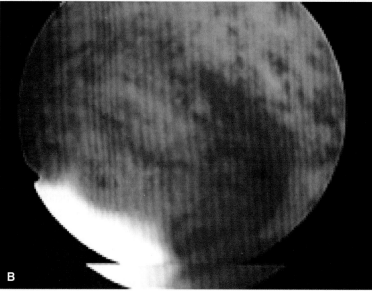

FIGURE 15.1.5 ● **A:** Hysteroscope being rotated to view the left cornu. **B:** Endoscopic view of left cornu and internal tubal meatus. From Berman JM, Shavell VI. Office hysteroscopy. In: Mayeaux EJ, ed. *The essential guide to primary care procedures.* Philadelphia, PA: Lippincott Williams & Wilkins, 2009.

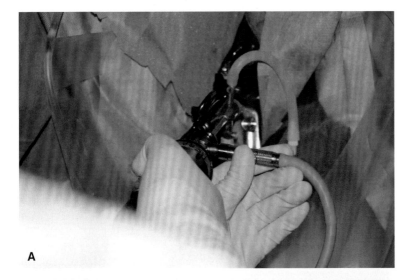

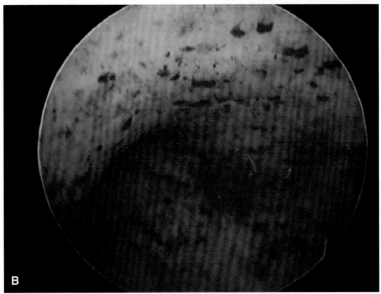

FIGURE 15.1.6 ● **A:** Hysteroscope rotated to view right aspect of endometrium. **B:** Endoscopic view of right uterine wall and tubal os. From Berman JM, Shavell VI. Office hysteroscopy. In: Mayeaux EJ, ed. *The essential guide to primary care procedures.* Philadelphia, PA: Lippincott Williams & Wilkins, 2009.

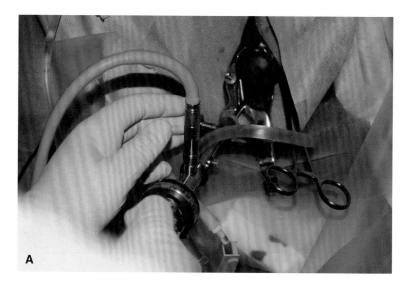

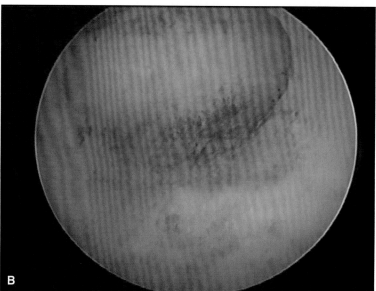

FIGURE 15.1.7 ● **A:** Hysteroscope rotated to view posterior aspect of endometrium.
B: Endoscopic view of posterior uterine wall and tubal os. From Berman JM, Shavell VI. Office hysteroscopy. In: Mayeaux EJ, ed. *The essential guide to primary care procedures.* Philadelphia, PA: Lippincott Williams & Wilkins, 2009.

AFTERCARE

- The patient may resume most normal activities within 24 hours.
- NSAIDs may be particularly useful for pain relief.

CPT Codes

58555. Hysteroscopy, diagnostic (separate procedure)
58558. Hysteroscopy, surgical; with sampling (biopsy) of endometrium and/or polypectomy, with or without D & C
58559. Hysteroscopy, surgical; with lysis of intrauterine adhesions (any method)
58560. Hysteroscopy, surgical; with division or resection of intrauterine septum (any method)
58561. Hysteroscopy, surgical; with removal of leiomyomata
58562. Hysteroscopy, surgical; with removal of impacted foreign body
58563. Hysteroscopy, surgical; with endometrial ablation (e.g., endometrial resection, electrosurgical ablation, thermoablation)
58565. Hysteroscopy, surgical; with bilateral fallopian tube cannulation to induce occlusion

PEARLS

- A zero-degree hysteroscope provides a "straight on" panoramic view in line with the sheath. Increasing viewing angles facilitates visualization of either side of midline, while minimizing side-to-side movement of the hysteroscope.
- Consider pretreatment with misoprostol 200 mcg buccally the night prior to procedure to soften the cervix, decrease pain associated with dilation, and to help overcome cervical stenosis. This works best in premenopausal women and is of questionable value in postmenopausal women.
- Consider pretreatment with NSAIDS the day prior to procedure to provide uterine quiescence, especially for women undergoing sterilization.
- For premenopausal women, the early proliferative phase is best for visualization of the uterine cavity, as thick secretory endometrium can obscure pathology and be misconstrued as endometrial polyps. Alternatively, place the patient on hormonal contraception by the beginning of the first day of the menstrual period preceding hysteroscopy.
- A minimum pressure for adequate visualization should always be used. This can usually be obtained under a maximum pressure of 75 to 100 mm Hg when using gravity or a hysteroscopic pump or a maximum CO_2 flow rate of 100 cc/min.
- CO_2 as a distension medium is generally reserved for diagnostic hysteroscopy.

Saline Infusion Sonohysterography

Brooke E. Friedman, Leah Millheiser, and
Paul D. Blumenthal

Saline infusion sonohysterography involves injecting saline into the uterine cavity transcervically under transvaginal ultrasound guidance. This procedure provides improved visualization of the endometrial lining, yielding better detection, and localization of endometrial pathology, such as submucosal leiomyomata or polyps.

RELEVANT ANATOMY (Fig. 15.2.1)

PATIENT POSITION

- The patient should be in the dorsal lithotomy position with her feet in stirrups.

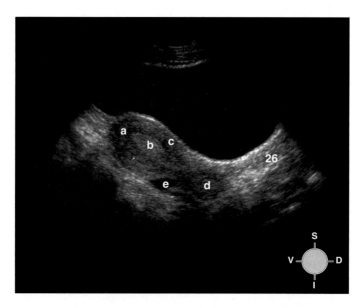

FIGURE 15.2.1 ● Sagittal view of female pelvis on ultrasound without saline infusion. (Key: S, superior; D, dorsal; I, inferior; V, ventral.) Radiographic key: (26) Vagina, (**a**) Myometrium, (**b**) Endometrium, (**c**) Uterus, (**d**) Cervix, (**e**) Fluid in retrouterine pouch (normal). From Dean D, Herbener TE. *Cross-sectional human anatomy.* Baltimore, MD: Lippincott Williams & Wilkins, 2000.

LANDMARKS

• The cervix must be visualized with a speculum.

ANESTHESIA

• Patients should be premedicated with ibuprofen 30 minutes prior to the procedure for pain control.
• There is no anesthesia necessary. A paracervical block may be used, however, for those patients with low pain tolerance or for those who experience significant cramping at the beginning of the procedure.

EQUIPMENT (Fig. 15.2.2)

• Ultrasound machine with transvaginal probe
• Sterile saline

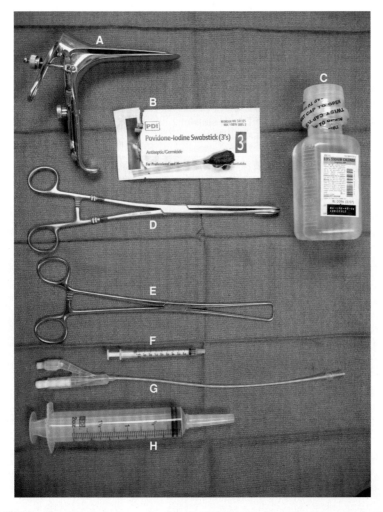

FIGURE 15.2.2 ● Sonohysterography tray. **A:** Graves or Pederson speculum, **B:** Povidone–iodine swabs, **C:** 0.9% normal saline, **D:** Ring forceps, **E:** Single-toothed tenaculum, **F:** Tuberculin syringe, **G:** Hysterosonographic catheter with two parts: (1) 3-cc balloon and (2) infusion part, **H:** 20-CL syringe.

- 60-cc syringe and 1-cc syringe
- Povidone–iodine solution
- Sonohysterography catheter
- Long ring forceps
- Single-tooth tenaculum (optional)
- Tape

TECHNIQUE

1. Insert the speculum into the vagina and visualize cervix.
2. Cleanse the cervix with a povidone–iodine solution, using a long ring forceps with soaked sponges or preprepared swabs.
3. Flush the sonohysterography catheter with sterile saline to purge it of air and minimize the risk of echogenic artifact.
4. Test the sonohysterogram balloon prior to placement of the catheter.
5. Guide the sonohysterography catheter into the cervix up to the fundus, using a sterile technique, with a long ring forceps (Fig. 15.2.3).
6. Inflate catheter balloon with 1 cc of sterile saline.
7. Remove stylet from catheter.
8. Tape catheter to thigh.
9. Remove speculum.
10. Insert the transvaginal ultrasound probe into the vagina (Fig. 15.2.4).
11. Attach a 60-cc syringe filled with sterile saline to the catheter.

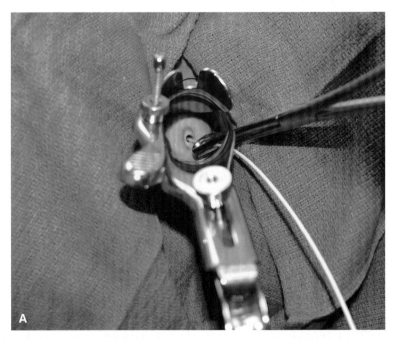

FIGURE 15.2.3 ● Insertion of catheter into cervix. **A:** Catheter being placed into cervix using ring forceps.

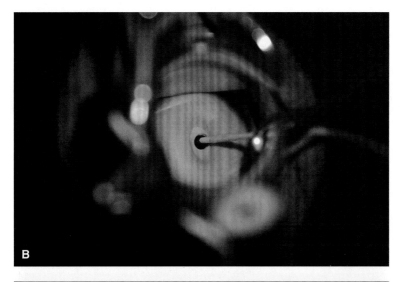

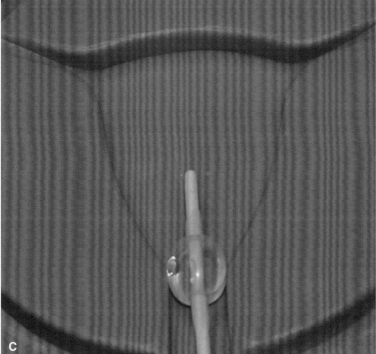

FIGURE 15.2.3 *(Continued)* ● **B:** Close-up of catheter being placed into cervix **C:** Correct placement of catheter in uterus with balloon deployed at internal cervical os.

12. Infuse saline while moving the probe from side-to-side and up-and-down to visualize the entire uterine cavity in both the coronal and sagittal views (Fig. 15.2.5).
13. Document findings either digitally or by printing out appropriate images during the procedure. The patient may also be shown the findings during the procedure by turning the ultrasound screen toward her.
14. Deflate the balloon, and remove the catheter and all instruments from the vagina.

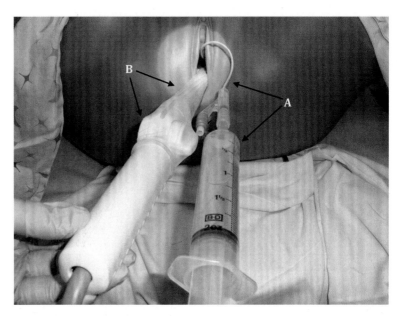

FIGURE 15.2.4 ● **A:** Sonohysterographic catheter being inserted into the vagina and cervical os. **B:** Ultrasound transducer being inserted into the vagina keeping pressure posterior to avoid discomfort.

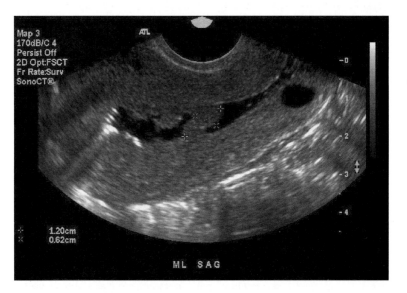

FIGURE 15.2.5 ● Sagittal view after saline infusion. Multiple small endometrial polyps noted after saline infusion. These polyps were not appreciated on transvaginal ultrasound (TVUS) without infusion. The anterior–posterior (A–P) measurement prior to infusion was 4.5 mm. From Baggish MS, Valle RF, Guedj H. *Hysteroscopy: visual perspectives of uterine anatomy, physiology and pathology.* Philadelphia, PA: Lippincott Williams & Wilkins, 2007.

AFTERCARE

- The patient can return to normal activities immediately after the procedure.
- NSAIDs may be helpful for any residual discomfort.

CPT Code
  958340.   Sonohysterography

PEARLS

- Schedule the procedure early in the follicular phase of the cycle, when the endometrial lining is thin to better visualize abnormalities.
- A single-tooth tenaculum may be used to stabilize the cervix while inserting the catheter.
- If cervical stenosis is encountered, cervical dilation may be necessary.
- If unable to achieve adequate uterine distension, the cervix may be overdilated. One can try to overcome this by placing ring forceps around the external cervical os.
- After deflating the balloon, continue infusing saline and observe uterine cavity from the exocervix to the fundus while removing the balloon.

Surgical Methods of Pregnancy Termination

Carrie Frederick and Paul D. Blumenthal

Surgical termination of pregnancy in the first trimester can be performed in office or procedure room settings. Oral analgesics may be used, or, given appropriate equipment for monitoring and administration, IV narcotics and/or tranquilizers. Aspiration using either manual or electrically generated vacuum is the most common approach.

First Trimester (up to 14 weeks of gestation)

RELEVANT ANATOMY (Fig. 16.1.1A,B)

PATIENT POSITION

- Lithotomy position

ANESTHESIA

Local Anesthesia

- Paracervical block using 10 to 20 mL 1% lidocaine (see Chapter 13.7, Paracervical Block)

Oral Analgesia

- Hydrocodone/Acetaminphen 5/500 1 to 2 tabs (or similar) PO +/− Valium 10 mg PO 1 hour before procedure

Moderate Sedation

- Versed 1 to 3 mg IV followed by Fentanyl 50 to 100 mcg IV before beginning procedure

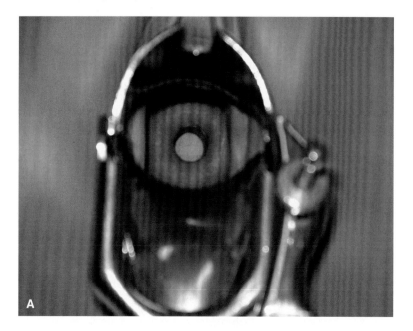

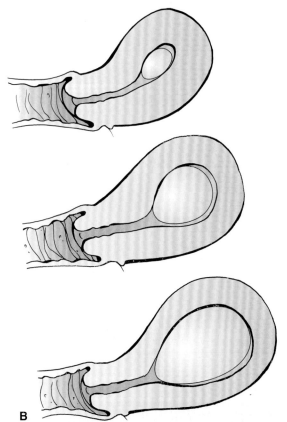

FIGURE 16.1.1 ● **A:** A clear view of the cervix through the speculum is important for expeditious care. **B:** Sagittal view of pregnancy in early, mid, and late first trimester. From Pillitteri A. *Maternal and child nursing,* 4th ed. Philadelphia, PA: Lippincott Williams & Wilkins, 2003.

EQUIPMENT

- Vaginal speculum (preferably Graves, Collins, or Klopfer)
- Tenaculum (single-toothed or atraumatic vulsellum forceps)
- Ring forceps
- 4 × 4 sponges
- Set of sequential cervical dilators (Pratt [preferable] or Hegar)
- Electric or manual vacuum aspiration device (Fig. 16.1.2A,B)

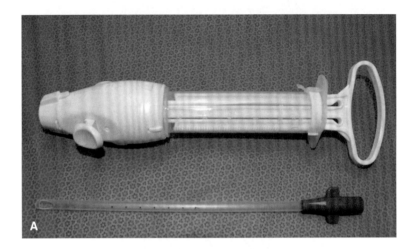

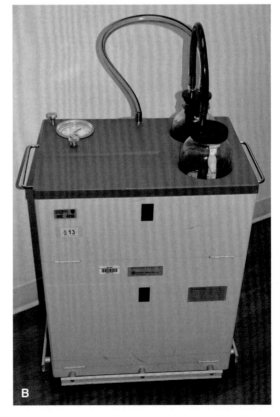

FIGURE 16.1.2 ● Aspiration Equipment. **A:** Manual vacuum aspiration (MVA) syringe with typical flexible suction canula. **B:** Electric vacuum aspiration (EVA) unit.

- Suction cannulae of various sizes (5 to 14 mm diameter)—to determine optimal size to use, choose estimated gestational age in weeks and use that number or age in weeks minus 1 or 2 depending on pliability of cervix, patient pain tolerance, and gestational age. Smaller cannula size will likely require more "passes" into the uterus to complete the evacuation
- Tissue forceps
- Scissors (if using electric suction machine—necessary to remove collection sock form aspirator)
- Sterile bowl
- Sterile water (to assist on viewing villi in very early gestations)
- Strainer to wash and separate products of conception (POC) and distinguish villi from decidua

Other medications and treatments to have available

- Methergine
- Silver nitrate sticks
- Monsel's solution
- Misoprostol tablets
- Prostaglandin 15-methyl F2α (Hemabate)
- Foley or Bakri balloon

TECHNIQUE

Preparation

- Patient should be draped or instruments positioned such that the patient cannot see the procedure being performed or instruments being used, but so that eye contact with the operator can be maintained.
- Instruments and tissue should also be carefully kept out of the patient's line of sight.

PROCEDURE

1. Perform ultrasound to confirm gestational age (this can be done 1 or more days prior to the procedure if necessary or more convenient).
2. Perform bimanual examination to assess uterine size and position (anteverted, midposition, or retroverted).
3. Place folded sterile towels over perineum, and if possible, have a sterile shelf or basin just beneath patient's buttocks (Fig. 16.1.3).
4. Place speculum in vagina and cleanse entire vagina and cervix with Betadine solution or other antiseptic.
5. Inject 1 to 2 mL lidocaine on anterior or posterior lip of cervix at 6 or 12 o'clock position producing wheal that extends laterally across cervix.
6. Grasp anesthetized lip of cervix with tenaculum or vulsellum forceps (Fig. 16.1.4A,B).
7. Administer paracervical block (see Fig. 13.7.1, Chapter 13.7, Paracervical Block).
8. Gently dilate cervical canal as needed up to size required to accommodate the cannula to be used (to convert Pratt mm to equivalent Hegar dilator, divide number of mm by 3). Note: Dilator does not have to be inserted more than a centimeter or 2 past internal cervical os.

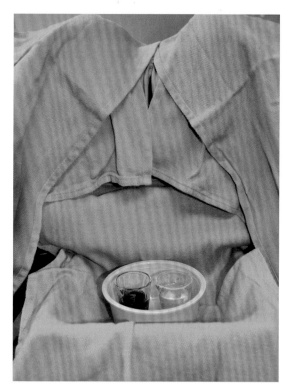

FIGURE 16.1.3 ● Draped "patient" showing drawer and basin below buttocks of patient, establishing a sterile work space in front of the operator.

9. Gently advance cannula into uterine cavity up to fundus, then withdraw slightly (Fig. 16.1.5).

10. Turn on suction machine/release valve on manual aspirator. Gently rotate cannula while progressively withdrawing to level of internal cervical os, until uterine cavity has gritty texture and appears to "grasp" or "grip" the cannula. No further tissue is seen passing through cannula and is replaced by bubbles or froth. Depending on cannula size and gestational age, several passes of this type may be necessary until POC are adequately evacuated and uterus contracts around cannula (Figs. 16.1.6 and 16.1.7).

11. Once entire uterine cavity feels gritty, remove cannula from uterus with suction off (i.e., close valves, release "slide mechanism" on suction tubing or turn off suction machine).

12. Inspect for bleeding from uterine cavity and cervical os.

13. If more than scant bleeding, consider an additional pass with the suction cannula.

14. If bleeding appears to be coming from cervix at tenaculum site, may use direct pressure with sponge stick, silver nitrate sticks, Monsel's solution, or suture as deemed necessary.

15. Inspect aspirated tissue to check for villi/placenta and fetal parts c/w gestational age (Fig. 16.1.8).

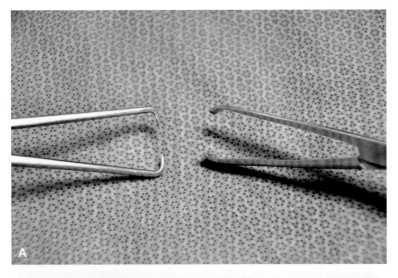

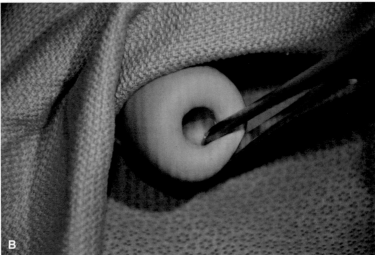

FIGURE 16.1.4 ● **A:** Comparative views of tenaculum tips. Conventional single-toothed tenaculum on left, and atraumatic vulsellum forceps (Shah) on right. **B:** Atraumatic vulsellum forceps (Shah) applied to cervix. Note that jaws of vulsellum forceps do not pierce cervical tissue.

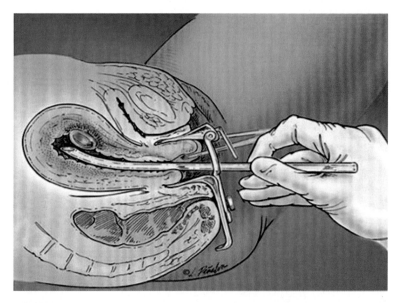

FIGURE 16.1.5 ● Suction cannula being inserted to uterine fundus. From Frankel N, Abernathy M, eds. *Performing uterine evacuation with the Ipas MVA Plus® aspirator and Ipas EasyGrip® cannulae: Instructional booklet,* 2nd ed. Chapel Hill, NC: Ipas, 2007.

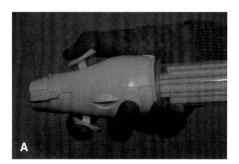
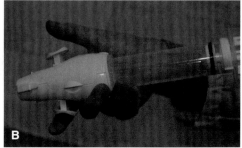

FIGURE 16.1.6 ● Valves on manual vacuum aspiration syringe being released, thus establishing vacuum to uterine cavity. **A:** Valves closed (buttons pressed forward and downward). Pulling the piston back "charges" the syringe. **B:** Valves released with syringe "charged", thus transmitting vacuum from uterus into syringe.

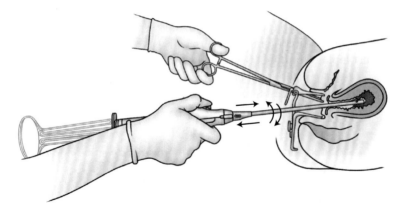

FIGURE 16.1.7 ● Rotating and curetting motion of cannula–syringe unit. From Frankel N, Abernathy M, eds. *Performing uterine evacuation with the Ipas MVA Plus® aspirator and Ipas EasyGrip® cannulae: Instructional booklet,* 2nd ed. Chapel Hill, NC: Ipas, 2007.

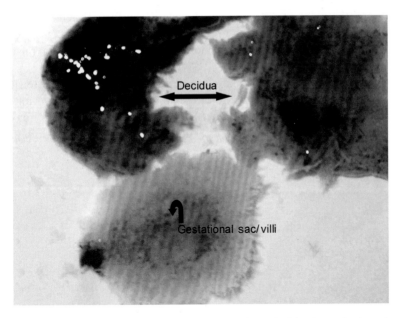

FIGURE 16.1.8 ● Gestational sac visible and distinct from decidua in washed specimen after manual vacuum aspiration.

CPT Codes

59840. Induced abortion (performed surgically)
59820. Missed abortion (completed surgically)
59812. Incomplete abortion (completed surgically)
76811. Transabdominal ultrasound with biometric measurements
76817. Transvaginal ultrasound

PEARLS

- Misoprostol 400 mcg buccal 2 hours prior to procedure can help prepare the cervix prior to procedure.
- Be sure to check Rh status and administer Rhogam if Rh negative.
- There is no need for a "check (sharp) curettage" if uterus is noted to be gritty to suction cannula, hemostasis is good, and the volume of POC is consistent with gestational age (including presence of fetal parts if gestational age is advanced enough to make them visible).
- Although traditionally the tenaculum has been placed horizontally across the anterior lip of the cervix, there are advantages to placing the tenaculum or vulsellum forceps "vertically" across the cervical os, with one blade of the instrument in the os itself and the other on the anterior or posterior surface. When placed this way: (1) Better cervical stabilization can be achieved since the actual cervix as opposed to vaginal mucosa is being grasped; (2) less bleeding is apparent when the speculum is removed.
- Irrespective of uterine position, there are advantages to placing the tenaculum or cervical stabilizer on the posterior lip of the cervix instead of the anterior lip: (1) It is easier to administer the paracervical block; (2) the tenaculum does not get in the way of the suction cannula or forceps, needing to constantly be held up and out of the way.

Second-trimester Dilation and Evacuation (14 through 23 weeks)

Carrie Frederick and Paul D. Blumenthal

While dilatation and evacuation can be performed in the office, training beyond first-trimester procedures is necessary in order to safely and expeditiously perform the procedure described below.

RELEVANT ANATOMY (Fig. 16.2.1)

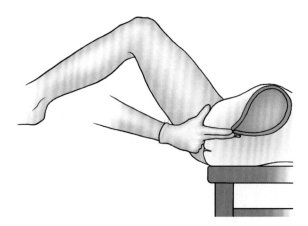

FIGURE 16.2.1 ● Sagittal view of pelvis showing relative size of second-trimester uterus. From Frankel N, Abernathy M, eds. *Performing uterine evacuation with the Ipas MVA Plus® aspirator and Ipas EasyGrip® cannulae: instructional booklet,* 2nd ed. Chapel Hill, NC: Ipas, 2007.

PATIENT POSITION

- Lithotomy position

LANDMARKS

- Same as for first-trimester procedure

ANESTHESIA

Local Anesthesia

- Paracervical block using 10 to 20 mL 1% lidocaine with 5 units vasopressin mixed with 20-cc lidocaine (see Chapter 13.7, Paracervical Block)

Oral Analgesia

- Hydrocodone/Acetaminphen 5/500 1 to 2 tabs (or similar) PO +/− Valium 10 mg PO 1 hour before procedure

Moderate Sedation

- Versed 1 to 3 mg IV followed by fentanyl 50 to 100 mcg IV before beginning procedure

EQUIPMENT

- Clean or sterile gloves
- Speculum
- Tenaculum or atraumatic vulsellum forceps (see Figure 16.1.4)
- Cannulae of various sizes
- Dilators
- Forceps (Fig. 16.2.2 Sopher, Bierer, etc.)

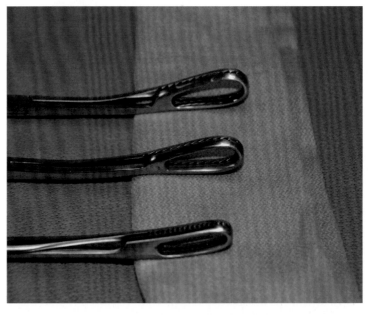

FIGURE 16.2.2 ● Forceps typically used in second-trimester dilatation and evacuation (D& E) procedures. The diameter of the tips of the largest **(top)** forceps is 19 mm, the smallest **(bottom)** is 14 mm.

- Large postpartum (Hunter's or "banjo") curette
- Sponges
- Local anesthetic
- Method of vacuum aspiration (manual or electric)

TECHNIQUE

Preparation

- Confirm gestational age of pregnancy with ultrasound
- Perform bimanual examination to assess size and position of uterus
- Prepare cervix with 600 µg misoprostol buccally 3 to 4 hours before procedure and place osmotic dilators such as laminaria or Dilapan™ the day prior (or in later gestational ages, a 2-day preparation may be required, with just a few devices placed on day 1, more devices added on day 2 [or much later in the day on day 1], and the procedure performed on day 2 (Fig. 16.2.3A,B)). Mifepristone, 200 mg orally, can also

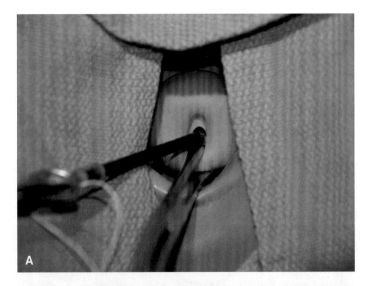

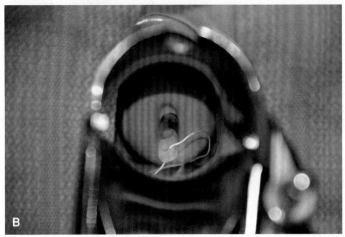

FIGURE 16.2.3 ● **A:** Osmotic dilator on ring forceps about to be inserted into cervix.
B: Single osmotic dilator properly seated in cervix.

be used to prepare cervix overnight, either in lieu of (14 to 19 weeks) or in addition to single set of cervical osmotic dilators (19 to 24 weeks).

D&E PROCEDURE

1. Begin in same fashion as with first-trimester procedure (steps 1 to 8 above). Key difference is that a speculum with a wider aperture than standard Graves (e.g., Collins, "wide body" Graves) is needed to ensure good visualization of cervix with adequate room for instrument manipulation (Fig. 16.2.4).

2. Dilate the cervix gently with series of tapered dilators, enough to accommodate size 12- to 16-mm cannula. If the cervix is adequately prepared, the operator should plan on using the largest cannula the cervix will accommodate. However, for procedures beyond 16 weeks, a 16-mm cannula is advised.

3. If cervix is not soft enough to easily accommodate dilators without need for significant force, do not perform procedure. Repeat cervical preparation with additional 600 μg misoprostol PV (if no blood present) or buccal.

4. Insert appropriate-sized cannula, attached to aspirator, through cervix into uterine cavity. Suction as for first-trimester procedure, rotating cannula during suction.

5. When no further fluid or tissue passes through cannula, turn off suction and remove cannula, being careful not to touch the cannula tip.

6. Hold forceps with third or fourth finger through the posterior ring, and the thumb against (but not in) the anterior ring (Fig. 16.2.5).

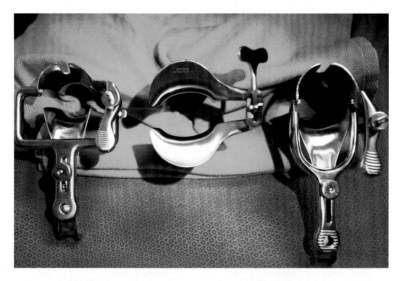

FIGURE 16.2.4 ● Different speculum types for second-trimester surgical abortion. Left to right, "Vu-more" speculum with extra wide aperture for instrumentation and access, Collins speculum with jaws that open in two dimensions given excellent view and access, standard Graves-style speculum with wider aperture for access and instrumentation.

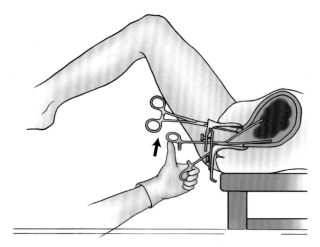

FIGURE 16.2.5 ● Forceps being opened in utero using correct orientation and hand position on forceps. From Frankel N, Abernathy M, eds. *Performing uterine evacuation with the Ipas MVA Plus® aspirator and Ipas EasyGrip® cannulae: instructional booklet,* 2nd ed. Chapel Hill, NC: Ipas, 2007.

7. Maintain firm but gentle traction on tenaculum and insert forceps through cervix. Once forceps blades pass through internal os, gently open the forceps as wide as necessary (Fig. 16.2.6A,B).
8. Use sonography to guide placement and location of instruments in uterus relative to location of fundus and fetal parts (Fig. 16.2.7).
9. Firmly grasp fetal tissue and withdraw forceps slowly while rotating forceps up to 90 degrees. When removing tissue, release tenaculum or vulsellum forceps and push gently against speculum for countertraction. Take particular care when removing calvarium and long bones of fetus as these carry additional risk of cervical laceration. Place tissue in sterile bowl.
10. Continue with forceps as above until confident all fetal and placental tissue has been removed.
11. Vacuum aspiration may be used at the end of procedure to gently remove any remaining tissue in uterine cavity—consider using smaller cannula such as 8- to 12-mm diameter, depending on gestational age.
12. Inspect fetal parts to confirm all are present and accounted for. Ultrasound can be used to confirm a thin endometrial stripe, indicating an empty uterus.
13. Inspect for bleeding and administer uterotonics as necessary.

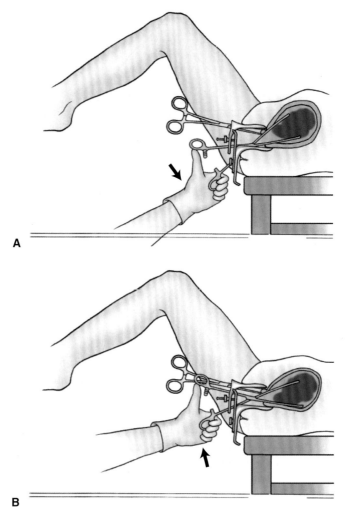

A

B

FIGURE 16.2.6 ● **A:** As forceps are inserted into the uterus the "heel" (held end) of the forceps is dropped posteriorly to allow the "toe" (tissue grasping end) to move anteriorly consonant with uterine position in most cases. From Frankel N, Abernathy M, eds. *Performing uterine evacuation with the Ipas MVA Plus® aspirator and Ipas EasyGrip® cannulae: instructional booklet,* 2nd ed. Chapel Hill, NC: Ipas, 2007. **B:** Forceps being closed and evacuating tissue from more central position in the uterus. From Frankel N, Abernathy M, eds. *Performing uterine evacuation with the Ipas MVA Plus® aspirator and Ipas EasyGrip® cannulae: instructional booklet,* 2nd ed. Chapel Hill, NC: Ipas, 2007.

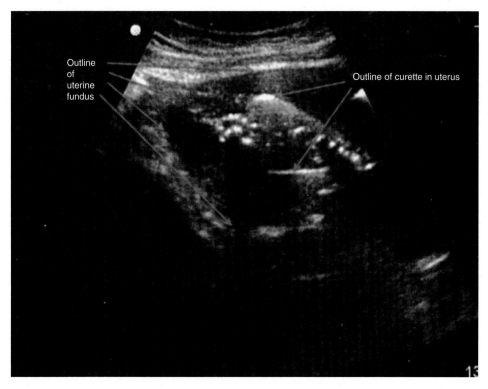

Outline of uterine fundus

Outline of curette in uterus

FIGURE 16.2.7 ● Intraoperative ultrasound image of large curette in uterus.

AFTERCARE

- If patient received analgesia/anesthesia, monitor until effects have worn off and ensure the woman has a ride home.
- Doxycycline 100 mg PO BID × 3 to 7 days
- Methergine 0.2 mg PO q8h × 2 days prn
- Motrin or other NSAIDs for pain/cramping
- Caution patient to monitor for fever >38.5° Celsius or bleeding that soaks a pad/h × 3 hours
- Contraception such as IUD or implant can be provided at the time of the procedure. Prescriptions can be written for oral contraceptives, vaginal ring, or patch. DMPA injection can also be given on the day of the abortion procedure.

CPT Codes

59841. Induced abortion, by dilation and evacuation
59200. Insertion of cervical dilator (eg, laminaria, prostaglandin) (separate procedure)
64435. Paracervical block
99144. Moderate sedation services provided by the same physician performing the diagnostic or therapeutic service that the sedation supports, requiring the presence of an independent trained observer to assist in the monitoring of the patient's level of consciousness and physiological status; age 5 years or older, first 30 minutes intra-service time
76815. Intraoperative transabdominal ultrasound

PEARLS

- Have optional instruments available to be able to manage minor complications such as cervical laceration, which may require suturing.
- Uterotonic agents such as misoprostol, oxytocin (if gestational age is greater than 18 weeks), 15-methyl Prostaglandin F2α, or methergine should be available in case of unexpected bleeding from uterine atony.
- Intravenous fluids (and the capacity to administer them) should also be available in case of severe bleeding to provide vascular support.

Intrauterine Insemination

Brooke E. Friedman and Mary T. Jacobson

Intrauterine insemination (IUI) bypasses the cervix and places concentrated sperm directly into the uterine cavity. IUI can be used to treat infertility resulting from different etiologies, such as sexual dysfunction, male factor, cervical factor, endometriosis, or unexplained infertility. IUI can be performed with a natural cycle, or with controlled ovarian hyperstimulation with clomiphene citrate, letrozole, or injectable gonadotropins.

RELEVANT ANATOMY (Fig. 17.1)

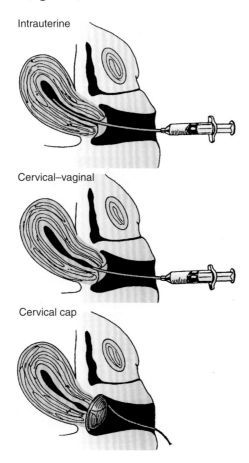

Intrauterine

Cervical–vaginal

Cervical cap

FIGURE 17.1 ● Techniques of artificial insemination. From Beckmann CR, Ling FW, et al. *Obstetrics and gynecology,* 5th ed. Philadelphia, PA: Lippincott Williams & Wilkins, 2006.

PATIENT POSITION

- The patient should lie on an examination table in dorsal lithotomy position with her feet in stirrups. It may be helpful for women with an anteverted uterus to maintain a full bladder to place the uterus in a more axial direction.

LANDMARKS

- The cervix must be visualized with a speculum.
- It may be helpful to have an assistant perform abdominal ultrasound guidance to visualize the uterine cavity during the procedure.

ANESTHESIA

- No anesthesia is needed

EQUIPMENT (Fig. 17.2)

- Prepared sperm specimen
- Speculum
- 1-cc sterile syringe
- Sterile blunt cannula or needle
- Disposable insemination catheter
- Rigid stylet for catheter (optional)
- Single-tooth tenaculum (optional)
- Ultrasound with abdominal probe (optional)

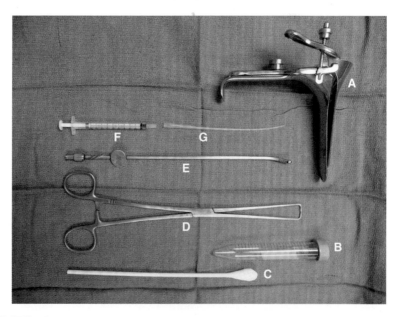

FIGURE 17.2 ● Insemination tray. **A:** Graves or Pederson speculum, **B:** Semen specimen container, **C:** Vaginal swab, **D:** Ring forceps, **E:** Novaks curette, **F:** Tuberculin syringe, and **G:** Semen insemination catheter.

TECHNIQUE

1. Confirm luteinizing hormone (LH) surge before proceeding with IUI. This can be done via over-the-counter ovulation predictor kits in natural cycles. Alternatively, with controlled ovarian hyperstimulation, one can monitor follicular development with a transvaginal ultrasound and administer a human chorionic gonadotropin (HCG) injection to trigger ovulation, when at least one follicle has reached a mean diameter of 15 to 18 mm. After a patient documents a positive morning LH surge with an ovulation predictor kit, IUI should be scheduled for 12 to 24 hours later. If an HCG trigger injection is used, IUI should be scheduled between 12 and 36 hours later.
2. At the appropriate scheduled time, collect fresh or frozen ejaculate for IUI processing (sperm processing and insemination techniques will not be described in this chapter).
3. Reconfirm the proper identification of both the patient and sperm sample in the laboratory and in the clinic. Reconfirm specific serum virology results of both the patient and sperm sample.
4. Aspirate approximately 0.5 mL of air into a 1-cc sterile syringe.
5. Attach a sterile cannula to the syringe and aspirate the processed sperm.
6. Attach the syringe to the insemination catheter.
7. Insert the speculum to visualize the cervix.
8. Use a cotton swab to wipe off any mucus from the cervical os.
9. Insert the catheter through the cervical os into the uterine cavity.
10. To facilitate a difficult catheter insertion, use a tenaculum on the cervix, a rigid stylet for the catheter, or abdominal ultrasound guidance (Fig. 17.3).

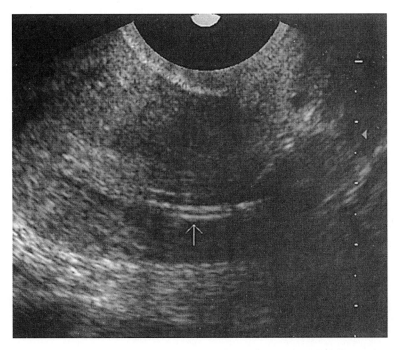

FIGURE 17.3 ● Ultrasound demonstrating an echogenic insemination catheter in the endometrial canal. From Baggish MS, Valle RF, Guedj H. *Hysteroscopy: visual perspectives of uterine anatomy, physiology and pathology.* Philadelphia, PA: Lippincott Williams & Wilkins, 2007.

11. Inject the sperm and then slowly withdraw the catheter.
12. Remove all instruments from the vagina.

AFTERCARE

- Allow the patient to rest in the supine position for 5 to 10 minutes after the procedure.
- The patient may resume her normal activities after insemination.
- Use Motrin for abdominal cramping or discomfort as needed.

CPT Code

58322.   Intrauterine insemination (IUI)

PEARLS

- Maintain the ejaculate specimen at body temperature until it is time for insemination.
- Do not use povidone–iodine to cleanse the cervix prior to insemination, as it is toxic to sperm.
- To minimize cramping and endometrial disruption, avoid touching the uterine fundus with the catheter at the time of insemination.

18

Trigger-point Injections: Abdomen, Buttocks, and Skin

Thuong-Thuong Nguyen, Paul D. Blumenthal, and Mary T. Jacobson

Trigger points are focal, nodular areas of hyperirritability within a taut band of skeletal muscle. They are tender to palpation and can lead to muscular twitching and referred pain to other sites. Trigger points are commonly found in the neck, shoulders, and pelvic girdle. Treatment techniques include application of ice or heat, physical therapy, acupuncture or acupressure, the Spray and Stretch technique using cooling Fluori-Methane or ethyl-chloride, transcutaneous electrical nerve stimulation (TENS), dry needling, radiofrequency treatment, and "trigger-point" injections of anesthetics, steroids, alcohol, or Botulinum toxin. Of these options, trigger-point injections are a more effective method of providing immediate, symptomatic relief from trigger-point pain.

Contraindications

- Known bleeding disorders or anticoagulation therapy
- Aspirin taken within 3 days of injection
- Acute muscle trauma
- Acute infection in site of injection or systemically
- Fear of needles
- Cellulitis or other evidence of acute infection at site of planned injection

RELEVANT ANATOMY: Common trigger points (Fig. 18.1 A–D)

PATIENT POSITION

- Supine, prone, or dorsolithotomy depending upon injection site

LANDMARKS

Landmarks depend on location of trigger point. Procedure for injection describes "trigger point" itself, and, in turn, that becomes the landmark.

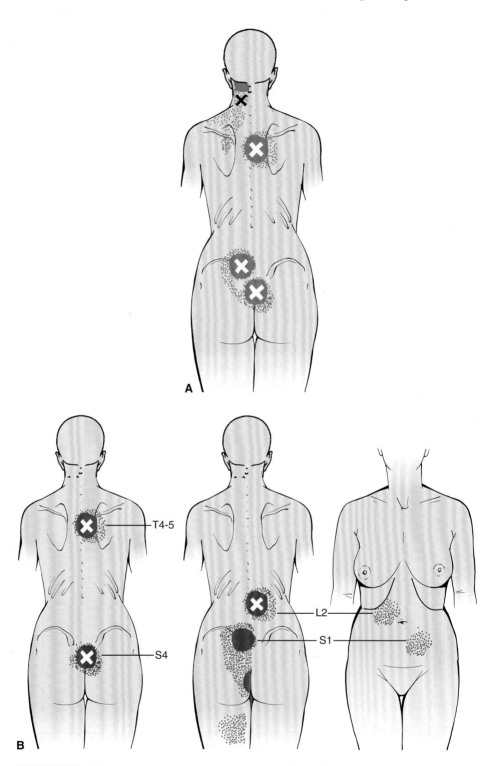

FIGURE 18.1 ● **A–D:** Common trigger points. **A:** Myofascial pain syndrome: Trigger points and referred pain patterns. **B:** Rotatores and multifidi m., trigger points. Referred pain pattern of trigger points (Xs) in deep paraspinal muscles (multifidi and rotaries). Solid red shows essential referred pain zone. Stippling maps spillover zone. MediClip image copyright © 2012 Lippincott Williams & Wilkins. All rights reserved.

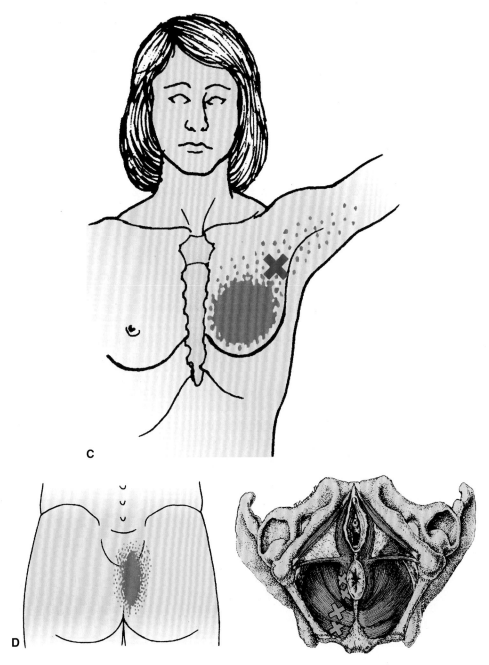

FIGURE 18.1 *(Continued)* ● **C:** Pectoralis major m., trigger points. Referred pain pattern with location of trigger point (X) for lateral free margin of left pectoralis major muscle. Solid red shows essential referred pain zone. Stippling maps spillover zone. MediClip image copyright © 2012 Lippincott Williams & Wilkins. All rights reserved. **D:** Pelvic musculature. Referred pain pattern of trigger points (Xs) in right sphincter ani, levator ani, and coccygeus muscles. Solid red shows essential referred pain zone. Stippling maps spillover zone. MediClip image copyright © 2012 Lippincott Williams & Wilkins. All rights reserved.

EQUIPMENT

- 21- to 27-gauge needle with length depending on site of injection
  - 1.5 inch to reach superficial muscles, 2 inch for gluteus maximus or paraspinal muscles, 2.5 inch for deeper gluteus minimus and quadrates lumborum muscles; pudendal nerve kit for transvaginal injection of pudendal nerve (see Chapter 10, Pudendal Block)
- 20- to 50-cc syringe
- Gloves
- Alcohol pads
- Gauze
- 1% Lidocaine, 0.25% bupivacaine, or 1% procaine without epinephrine
- Adhesive bandage

TECHNIQUE

1. Identify the trigger point and outline the borders by centering it between the index and middle fingers (Fig. 18.2). The pressure from the fingers will also help stabilize the trigger point for injection and minimize bleeding.
2. Clean the area with alcohol.
3. Insert the needle at a 30-degree angle 1 to 2 cm away from the trigger point.
4. Advance the needle toward the trigger point while maintaining the 30-degree angle.
   a. The patient may feel a pinching or twitching sensation.
5. Aspirate to ensure the needle is not in a blood vessel.
6. Inject 0.2 cc of anesthetic into the trigger point.
7. Withdraw the needle to the subcutaneous tissue.
8. Redirect the needle toward one quadrant of the point, advance, and inject another 0.2 cc.

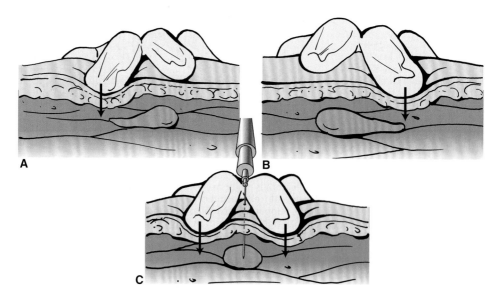

FIGURE 18.2 ● **A** and **B:** Localizing the trigger point between the index and the middle finger. **C:** Stabilizing trigger point and inserting needle for injection. Adapted from Alvarez DJ, Rockwell P. Trigger Points: Diagnosis and Management. *Am Fam Physician* 2002;65(4):653–661.

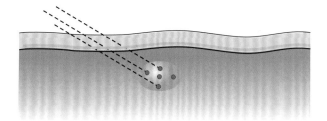

FIGURE 18.3 ● Superior, inferior, and medial or lateral aspects of trigger point are targets of injection. From Mayeaux EJ Jr. Trigger point injection. In: Mayeaux EJ Jr., ed. *The essential guide to primary care procedures*. Philadelphia, PA: Lippincott Williams & Wilkins, 2009: 898–903.

9. Repeat the process until injections have been made superiorly, inferiorly, medially, and laterally and continuing until there is palpable relaxation of the muscle (Fig. 18.3).
10. Palpate the area for further points of tenderness; then treat with injection.
11. Apply pressure to the injection site for 2 minutes.
12. Apply bandage.
13. Have the patient stretch and move the injected muscle group to increase injection efficacy.

COMPLICATIONS

- Hematoma development
- Infection
- Vasovagal syncope
- Needle breakage

AFTERCARE

- Postinjection soreness is common and resolves in 3 to 4 days.
- Advise the patient to avoid strenuous activity for 3 to 4 days.
- Repeat injection is not recommended until soreness resolves.

CPT Codes
20552. Trigger-point injection (one or two muscles)
20553. Trigger-point injection (three or more muscles)

PEARLS

- If, during the injection, the patient describes a sharp, electric pain extending locally and usually distally, the needle may have entered, or be very close to a nerve. To avoid possible injury or damage to the nerve, withdraw the needle and reposition the needle further away from the trigger point.

19

Hysteroscopic Sterilization (Essure)

Carrie Frederick and Mary T. Jacobson

Hysteroscopic sterilization can be performed in the office setting with minimal or no anesthesia and is an appropriate option for women who desire sterilization without the need for general anesthesia, or for women with comorbidities that confer unacceptable risk for abdominal or laparoscopic approaches.

Contraindications

- Pregnancy or suspected pregnancy
- Less than 6 weeks postpartum or postabortion
- Uncertain about permanent sterilization
- Active or recent pelvic infection
- Abnormal uterine or tubal anatomy that precludes access to tubal ostia
- Known allergy to contrast media (unable to perform hysterosalpingogram to confirm successful tubal occlusion)

Key Components of Counseling

- Sterilization is permanent
- Alternative contraceptive methods, including vasectomy
- Reasons for selecting sterilization
- Details of procedure, risks, and benefits
  - Risks include those associated with hysteroscopy, such as fluid overload, infection and cervical injury, as well as uterine or tubal perforation by hysteroscope or Essure device, insert expulsion, cramping, pain, nausea and/or vomiting, dizziness and/or light-headedness, and vaginal bleeding or spotting.
- Risk of failure and unilateral tubal occlusion
  - Risk of pregnancy after Essure procedure approximately 1/1,000; 5-year efficacy of 99.74%
  - Reasons for failure include pregnancy at time of placement, incorrect placement, noncompliance with postprocedure instructions and incorrect reading of hysterosalpingogram confirming tubal occlusion
- Risk of regret
  - Higher in women <30 years old undergoing sterilization, regardless of parity or marital status

- Sterilization does not protect against sexually transmitted infections
- Regulations (if applicable) mandating time interval from consent to procedure
- Need for a backup contraceptive method for a minimum of 12 weeks following procedure while tubal fibrosis occurs and hysterosalpingogram confirms tubal occlusion
- Essure microinserts may conduct electricity; therefore procedures using electrocautery such as endometrial ablation should be undertaken with caution in future
- Theoretical risks to pregnancy with Essure in situ, that is, nickel is a known mutagen and carcinogen

ANESTHESIA

- No anesthesia required
- If anesthesia preferred, paracervical block with 20-mL 1% lidocaine may be adequate (see Chapter 14.7, Paracervical Block)
- NSAIDS beginning 1 day prior to the procedure
- If patient is unable to tolerate procedure, moderate sedation may be used

EQUIPMENT

- 5-mm rigid hysteroscope with 5F operating channel
- 12- to 30-degree lens
- Hysteroscopic grasper
- Electrolyte solution, e.g., normal saline, for uterine distention
- Essure insertion device with two individually wrapped Essure devices (one for each tube) (Fig. 19.1). Have second package as back up in case of instrument malfunction or contamination.

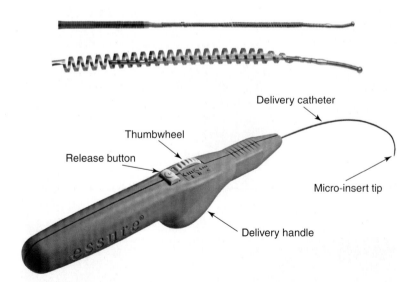

FIGURE 19.1 ● Unexpanded Essure microinsert **(top)**, expanded microinsert **(below)**, and insertion device with deliver handle **(bottom)**. Copyright © 2012 Conceptus Inc.

PRE-PROCEDURE

- Tubal ostia are easiest to visualize if endometrium is thin; may pretreat with combined hormonal contraception or a progestin or perform procedure after menses during early proliferative phase.
- Day prior to procedure, patient should take oral NSAIDs such as ibuprofen 600 mg by mouth every 6 hours.
- Single dose of misoprostol 200 to 400 mcg buccally or vaginally for cervical preparation (if indicated) night before procedure.
- Day of procedure, confirm a negative urine pregnancy.

TECHNIQUE

1. Perform a bimanual examination.
2. Insert either a side-opening or weighted speculum with a right angle retractor to elevate the anterior vaginal wall.
3. Prep the cervix with Betadine or other bacteriostatic agent.
4. Perform a paracervical block.
5. Grasp anterior or posterior lip of cervix with a tenaculum.
6. Gently dilate cervix to accommodate 5-mm hysteroscope.
7. Gently introduce hysteroscope and distend the uterine cavity with saline at a minimum infusion pressure for optimal visualization of the tubal ostia and placement of the inserts.
8. Confirm that both tubal ostia are visible and appear to be patent (if not, abort procedure). (see Chapter 15.1, Office Hysteroscopy, Figure 15.1.4)
9. Guide the Essure introducer through operating channel of hysteroscope into tubal lumen until black marker is at tubal orifice or when 5 to 10 mm of the proximal end of the microinsert is visible at the ostium (Fig. 19.2).

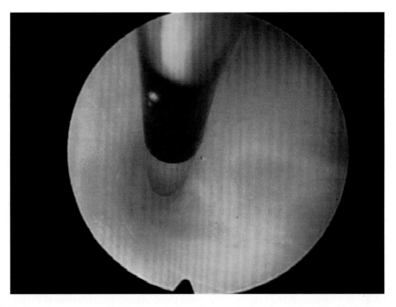

FIGURE 19.2 ● Essure system being deployed into tubal ostium with "black marker" indicating proper depth. From Berman JM. Hysteroscopic female sterilization. In: Mayeaux EJ, ed. *The essential guide to primary care procedures*. Philadelphia, PA: Lippincott Williams & Wilkins, 2009.

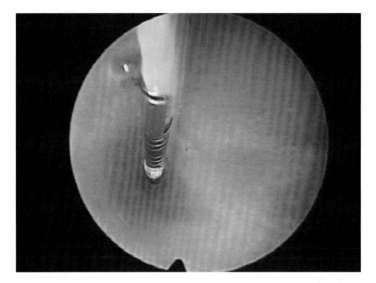

FIGURE 19.3 ● Essure coil being deployed from hysteroscope. Gold band is at level of tubal ostium. From Berman JM. Hysteroscopic female sterilization. In: Mayeaux EJ, ed. *The essential guide to primary care procedures.* Philadelphia, PA: Lippincott Williams & Wilkins, 2009.

10. Withdraw the hydrophilic outer cannula by rotating dial on Essure handpiece toward yourself until it will no longer rotate.
11. To confirm that insert is placed correctly, check that gold band "notch" is visible just outside ostium (Fig. 19.3).
12. Press deployment button. Rotate thumbwheel again toward yourself to detach device from delivery cannula.
    Three to eight coils should be visible trailing into uterine cavity (Fig. 19.4). If there are 18 or more coils visible, remove microinsert and re-attempt insertion with new device. Record number of coils visible.

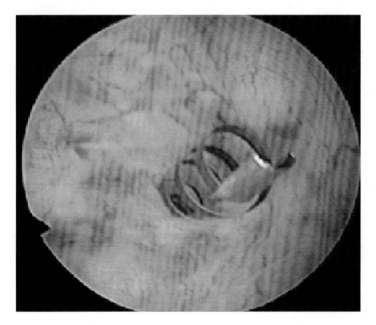

FIGURE 19.4 ● Essure coils protruding appropriately into endometrial cavity. Copyright © 2012 Conceptus Inc.

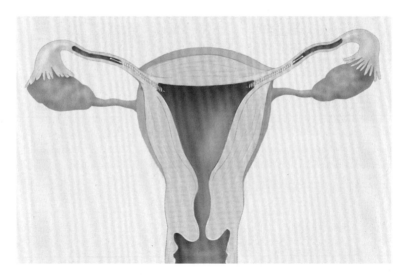

FIGURE 19.5 ● Schematic representation of completed Essure procedure with coils appropriately protruding from tubal meatus bilaterally. Copyright © 2012 Conceptus Inc.

13. Remove delivery cannula.
14. Repeat procedure for opposite tube. At end procedure, coils should be deployed as depicted schematically in Figure 19.5.

AFTERCARE

• Advise patient to call for fever, excessive vaginal bleeding, or severe or persistent pain.
• Perform hysterosalpingogram 3 months after placement to confirm tubal occlusion.
• Until hysterosalpingogram confirming bilateral tubal occlusion is performed, patient must use a backup form of contraception.

CPT Codes

58565. Hysteroscopy, surgical; with bilateral fallopian tube cannulation to induce occlusion by placement of permanent implants
58340. Postplacement test of tubal occlusion: Catheterization and introduction of saline or contrast material for hysterosalpingogram

PEARLS

• Perform procedure in the early proliferative phase of the endometrium or prep the endometrium with contraceptive hormones beginning the first day of the last menstrual period of the cycle of the scheduled procedure to optimize visualization.
• Use NSAIDS beginning 1 day prior to procedure to assist with uterine and tubal quiescence.
• IM or IV ketorolac decreases tubal spasm and may improve insertion success rates.

20

Contraceptive Procedures: Subdermal Contraceptive Implants

Thuong-Thuong Nguyen and Paul D. Blumenthal

Progesterone-releasing subdermal contraceptive devices, such as the Implanon, Jadelle, and Sinoplant-2, provide effective contraception for up to 3 to 5 years.

Devices

- **Implanon:** Duration: 3 years. Number of rods: One, ethylene vinyl acetate. Size: 4 cm long, 0.2 cm diameter. Progestin released: 68 mg of etonogestrel at a rate of 60 to 70 mcg/day initially, 35 to 45 mcg/day at the end of the first year, 30 to 40 mcg/day at the end of the second year, and finally 25 to 30 mcg/day at the end of the third year. Quoted rate of pregnancies: Pearl Index of 0.38 pregnancies per 100 women-years of use. Onset of effective contraception: Within 24 hours of insertion. Return of fertility after removal of rod: Quickly. Common side effect: Irregular bleeding. Availability: US and elsewhere. Training required by manufacturer: Yes (Fig. 20.1A).
- **Jadelle:** Duration: 5 years. Number of rods: Two. Size: 4.3 cm long, 0.25 cm diameter. Progestin released: 75 mg of levonorgestrel per rod at a rate of 80 mcg/day in the first month, 50 mcg/day by 9 months, and then 25 to 30 mcg/day. Availability: Not marketed in the United States, but is available in many other countries. Cumulative pregnancy rate in clinical trials: 0.3% at 3 years, 1.1% at 5 years. Common side effect: Unscheduled bleeding (Fig. 20.1B).

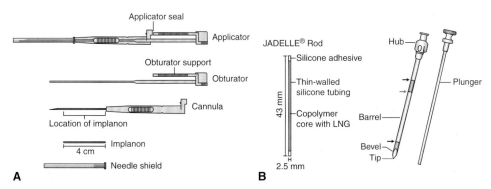

FIGURE 20.1 ● **A:** The Implanon system. Modified from and reproduced with permission of MSD Oss B.V., a subsidiary of Merck & Co., Inc., Whitehouse Station, New Jersey, USA. All rights reserved. NEXPLANON is a registered trademark of MSD Oss B.V. **B:** The Jadelle system. *(continued)*

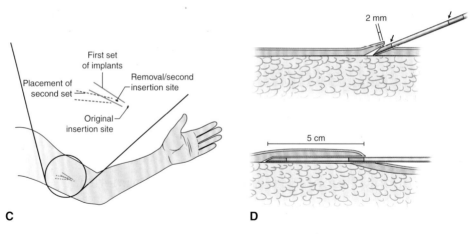

FIGURE 20.1 *(Continued)* ● **C** and **D**: Scheme for locating Jadelle insertion site **(C)** and insertion technique **(D)**. Permissions have been requested from Merck by Dr. Blumenthal. Tentatively granted and pending their final approval regarding colorized/rendered figures.

- Insertion is performed using local anesthesia. Using a no. 10 trocar (provided by the company), the rods are placed in a V configuration subdermally at the inner part of the nondominant upper arm. Removal is performed under local anesthesia by grasping the ends of the rods through a 3- to 4-mm incision at the apex of the V (Fig. 20.1C and D).
- **Sinoplant-2:** Similar to Jadelle, but only available in China, Indonesia, and other developing countries. Registered as "Zarin" in some countries.

Contraindications

- Pregnancy
- History of thrombotic or thromboembolic disorders
- History of breast cancer
- Liver disease
- Undiagnosed abnormal genital bleeding
- Allergies or sensitivities to implant components

Insertion of Implanon

EQUIPMENT (Fig. 20.2)

- A 25-gauge needle (1.5 inches long) attached to a 2- to 5-mL syringe
- 1% lidocaine without epinephrine
- Antiseptic solution: Betadine, chlorhexidine, and isopropyl alcohol
- Adhesive closure and bandage for puncture site
- Sterile surgical gloves
- Sterile drapes
- Sterile gauze
- Sterile disposable applicator preloaded with Implanon

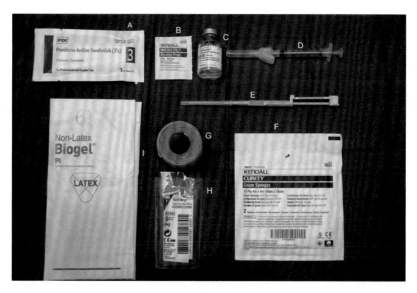

FIGURE 20.2 ⬤ Implanon tray. **A:** Povidone iodine swabs. **B:** Alcohol swabs. **C:** 1% Lido-caine solution **D:** 10-cc syringe with safety needle **E:** Implanon pre-loaded insertion device **F:** 4 × 4 gauze sponges **G:** wrap-type bandage for pressure dressing **H:** Steri-strips for insertion (or removal) site closure **I:** Sterile gloves.

PATIENT POSITION

- Supine: Nondominant arm rotated outward and bent at a 90-degree angle at the elbow, palm near patient's head. Arm should be well supported by the bed or table (Fig. 20.3).

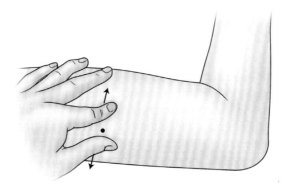

FIGURE 20.3 ⬤ Positioning arm in right-angle position. Modified from and reproduced with permission of MSD Oss B.V., a subsidiary of Merch & Co., Inc., Whitehouse Station, New Jersey, USA. All rights reserved. NEXPLANON is a registered trademark of MSD Oss B.V.

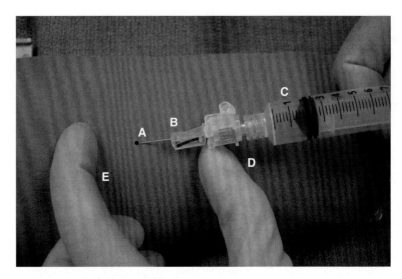

FIGURE 20.4 ● **A:** Skin marker placed where needle is to be injected. **B:** ≤22 gauge needle to provide subcutaneous anesthesia along the line of planned insertion. **C:** 10 cc syringe with 1% plain Lidocaine. 3 cc is sufficient. **D:** Thumb putting countertraction on skin. **E:** Index finger putting countertraction on skin in opposite direction.

LANDMARKS

- Identify the crease between the biceps and triceps muscles. This will be a groove in which the implant will be inserted.
- Mark the insertion site at 6 to 8 cm (or three fingerbreadths) superior and lateral to the medial epicondyle of the humerus.

ANESTHESIA

- Inject 1 to 2 cc of 1% lidocaine subcutaneously along the intended rod insertion track (Fig. 20.4 Implant local anesthesia).

TECHNIQUE

1. Confirm that the Implanon rod is in the needle. If it is not readily visible, point the applicator needle downward over a sterile field and tap the needle until the rod can be seen. Turning the applicator needle back upward and tapping the base on the table should then replace the rod into a position ready for insertion.
2. Remove the needle cover. Place the needle tip, bevel up, at the marked site of insertion (Fig. 20.5A). Pull the skin taut and push the needle and obturator directly through the skin at a 20-degree angle toward the patient's shoulder (Fig. 20.5B Trocar piercing skin image).
3. Once the needle is inserted, lower the angle of the needle until it is parallel to the skin (Fig. 20.5C and D).
4. Advance the needle within the subdermal tissue at this parallel angle while lifting or tenting the skin upward to avoid deep insertion of the needle (Fig. 20.5E Implant insertion tenting).

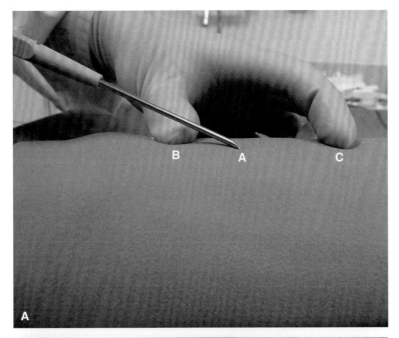

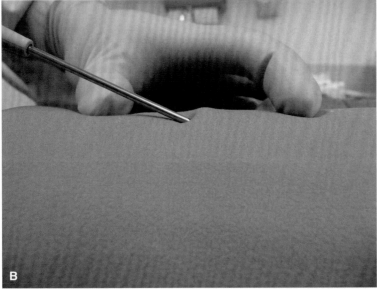

FIGURE 20.5 ● **A:** Implanon insertion: (A) Beveled end up, inserter is poised to break through the anesthetized skin and start subcutaneous track. (B) Thumb stabilizing skin with countertraction as trocar enters skin. (C) Index finger putting countertraction on skin in opposite direction. **B:** Trocar being introduced under the skin at a 20-degree angle. It is rapidly lowered and turned to enter the subdermal space parallel to the skin surface. Modified from and reproduced with permission of MSD Oss B.V., a subsidiary of Merch & Co., Inc., Whitehouse Station, New Jersey, USA. All rights reserved. NEXPLANON is a registered trademark of MSD Oss B.V. *(continued)*

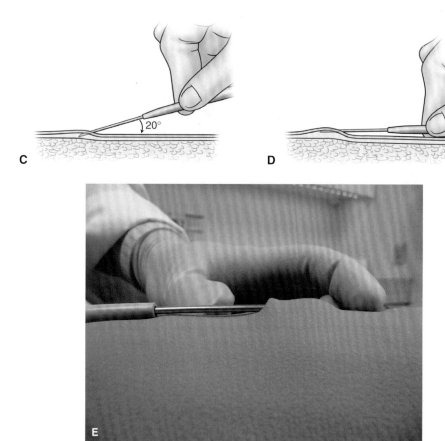

FIGURE 20.5 *(Continued)* ● **C:** Trocar piercing skin at 20-degree angle (cross-sectional view). Modified from and reproduced with permission of MSD Oss B.V., a subsidiary of Merck & Co., Inc., Whitehouse Station, New Jersey, USA. All rights reserved. NEXPLANON is a registered trademark of MSD Oss B.V. **D:** Trocar being positioned parallel to skin and advanced in subcutaneous space (cross-sectional view). Modified from and reproduced with permission of MSD Oss B.V., a subsidiary of Merck & Co., Inc., Whitehouse Station, New Jersey, USA. All rights reserved. NEXPLANON is a registered trademark of MSD Oss B.V. **E:** Trocar intermittently "tenting" skin and subcutaneous tissue on to upper mark.

5. Once the needle is advanced fully, press on the obturator support to break the applicator seal (Fig. 20.6A).
6. Turn the obturator 90 degrees with respect to the needle (Fig. 20.6B).
7. Stabilize the obturator with one hand, keeping the rod in place, and slowly withdraw the needle from the patient's arm (Fig. 20.6C Tenting crop image).
8. Confirm the rod is in place by palpating for both ends underneath the skin. If the rod is not palpable, examine the needle, which should reveal the grooved tip of the obturator. Confirmation can also be done by ultrasound (Fig. 20.6D).
9. Cover puncture site with adhesive closure and bandage.
10. Place the patient chart label in her medical record and give the patient her user card.

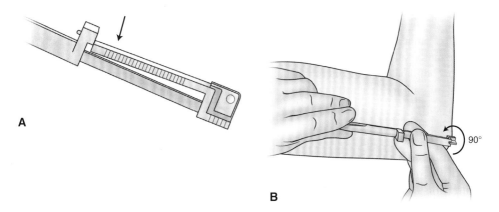

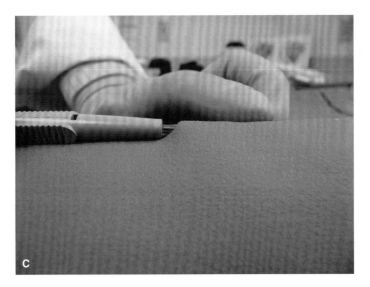

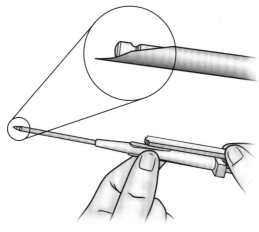

FIGURE 20.6 ● **A** and **B:** Inserter being prepared for release (**A**) and deposit of implant (**B**). Modified from and reproduced with permission of MSD Oss B.V., a subsidiary of Merch & Co., Inc., Whitehouse Station, New Jersey, USA. All rights reserved. NEXPLANON is a registered trademark of MSD Oss B.V. **C:** Implanon trocar completely inserted, in position to release the rod and withdraw the sleeve. **D:** Implant insertion rod visible at needle bevel, indicating implant deposited in skin. Modified from and reproduced with permission of MSD Oss B.V., a subsidiary of Merck & Co., Inc., Whitehouse Station, New Jersey, USA. All rights reserved. NEXPLANON is a registered trademark of MSD Oss B.V.

Side Effects and Complications

- Most women do not experience significant pain during or after insertion. NSAIDs are usually sufficient for pain control.
- Rare complications are infection, allergic reaction, expulsion, hematoma formation, local migration of the rod over time, and medial antebrachial cutaneous nerve damage.

AFTERCARE

- Counsel the patient that she may experience mild swelling and bruising. She should notify her MD if she develops severe pain, swelling of the arm, discharge at the insertion site or fever.

Implanon Removal ("Pop out" Technique)

1. Identify location of rod in the arm.
2. Elevate and identify one end of the rod (usually the distal end) by pressing down on the opposite (usually the proximal) end. Use local anesthesia, 1% lidocaine, injecting 1 to 3 cc *underneath* the distal tip of the implant.
3. Using a no. 11 blade, make a small incision over the identified end. A 2-mm incision should be sufficient for Implanon removal. The skin can be stretched slightly with the mosquito forceps if necessary.
4. Begin by gently pushing the implant toward the incision with your fingertip until the tip is visible in the incision (Fig. 20.7).
5. When the implant is visible in the incision, wipe away any fibrous tissue covering the device, grasp the end with a sterile mosquito forceps, and remove the rod (Fig. 20.7).
6. Cover the incision site with adhesive closure and bandage.

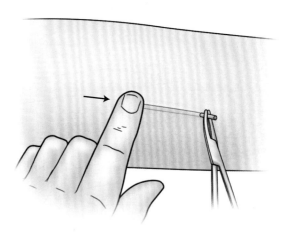

FIGURE 20.7 ● Implant being expressed toward incision and grasped with forceps. Modified from and reproduced with permission of MSD Oss B.V., a subsidiary of Merck & Co., Inc., Whitehouse Station, New Jersey, USA. All rights reserved. NEXPLANON is a registered trademark of MSD Oss B.V.

Implanon Removal (Instrument Technique)

Follow steps 1 to 5 above.

7. If the tip of the implant is not clearly visible, fibrous tissue may have formed around the implant. The fibrous tissue can be dissected away by continuing to cut toward the distal tip with the scalpel (Fig. 20.8A), until the tip is clearly visible. Remove the implant with forceps (Fig. 20.8B).
8. If the tip of the implant is still not visible, gently insert a forceps *into* the incision and grasp the implant (Fig. 20.8C), stabilizing it with the fingers of the other hand. With a second forceps carefully dissect the tissue around the implant. The implant can then be removed (Fig. 20.8D).

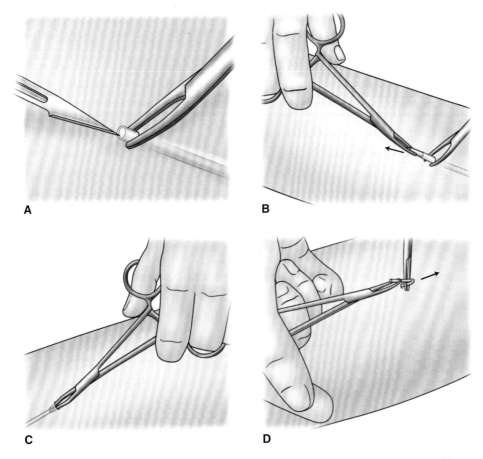

A   **B**

C   **D**

FIGURE 20.8 ● Instrument technique for implant removal. **A:** Scalpel used to dissect fibrous tissue sheath away from implant. **B:** Forceps used to remove implant after release from fibrous sheath. **C:** Forceps inserted *into* the incision to grasp implant subcutaneously and bring to incision. **D:** Second forceps used to grasp implant and remove, while first forceps stabilizes implant in incision. Modified from and reproduced with permission of MSD Oss B.V., a subsidiary of Merck & Co., Inc., Whitehouse Station, New Jersey, USA. All rights reserved. NEXPLANON is a registered trademark of MSD Oss B.V.

CPT Codes

11981. Insertion, non-biodegradable drug delivery implant
11982. Removal, non-biodegradable drug delivery implant

PEARLS

- Conditions requiring follow-up care: Diabetes, hypertension, depression, and headaches.
- Rifampin, some anticonvulsants, and some antiretroviral agents may make implants less effective, but even with slight reduction in effectiveness, implants will protect against pregnancy at a level comparable to other hormonal methods. Any medication the patient is taking should be checked for current information about drug–drug interactions with the implant.
- Implants may be placed at any time in the menstrual cycle (and placed immediately if switching from other form of contraception) and immediately postabortion or postpartum.
- If removal of rod(s) is difficult (i.e., rod[s] are not removed in 30 minutes), it may be better to stop the procedure for the client's comfort. In the event that the Implanon rod or both Jadelle/Sino-Implant (II) rods are not removed, ask the client to return when the incision site is fully healed (in about 4 to 6 weeks) and try again or refer to a more experienced clinician.

Note: Starting in 2012, the manufacturer of Implanon (Merck, Inc. Whitehouse Station, NJ) will be gradually replacing Implanon, with Nexplanon, an improved version of Implanon with the same drug content and a revised inserter. All the principles of Nexplanon insertion and removal are the same as with Implanon and in Figures 20.9A–C the essentials of insertion with the new inserter are displayed.

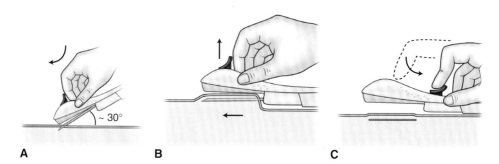

A   B   C

FIGURE 20.9 ● Nexplanon insertion. **A:** The skin is prepared as for Implanon and the Nexplanon inserter positioned above the insertion site at a 30-degree angle. **B:** The inserter is advanced subdermally as for Implanon until the hilt of the needle/trocar is reached. **C:** Keeping the applicator in the same position unlock the purple slider by pushing it slightly down. Move the slider fully back until it stops. The implant is now in its final subdermal position, and the needle is locked inside the body of the applicator. The applicator can now be removed. Modified from and reproduced with permission of MSD Oss B.V., a subsidiary of Merck & Co., Inc., Whitehouse Station, New Jersey, USA. All rights reserved. NEXPLANON is a registered trademark of MSD Oss B.V.

Intrauterine Contraception

Jessica Kassis and Paul D. Blumenthal

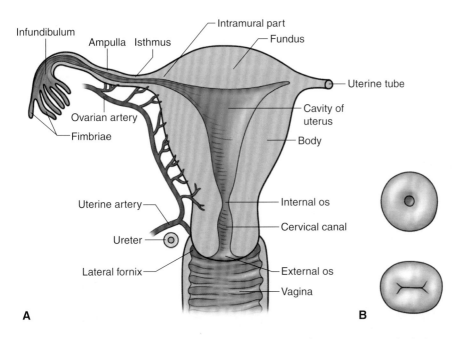

There are currently two intrauterine contraceptives (IUCs) available for use in the United States. These include the copper IUC (TCu380A, ParaGard) and a levonorgestrel-releasing IUC (LNg 20, Mirena). Prior to insertion of an IUC, it is important to discuss the advantages, disadvantages, and common side effects associated with the chosen IUC. In addition, written consent should be obtained. One should also exclude any conditions precluding IUC placement, including possible or confirmed pregnancy, recent or recurrent uterine infection, active genital actinomycoses, untreated cervicitis, or distortion of the uterine cavity.

RELEVANT ANATOMY (Fig. 21.1)

PATIENT POSITION

- Lithotomy position

FIGURE 21.1 ● **A–D:** Pelvic anatomy demonstrating route of IUD insertion and relative uterine positions. Modified from Michael S. Baggish, Rafael F. Valle, Hubert Guedj. *Hysteroscopy: Visual Perspectives of Uterine Anatomy, Physiology and Pathology.* Philadelphia, PA: Lippincott Williams & Wilkins, 2007. *(continued)*

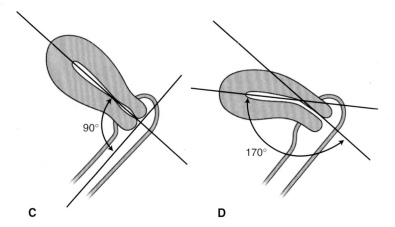

FIGURE 21.1 *(Continued)*

LANDMARKS

- See Figure 21.1
- With speculum in place, cervix must be visualized.

ANESTHESIA

- Although not required, a paracervical block prior to IUC insertion can be administered. (See Chapter 13.7.) This involves the injection of 10 to 20 cc of 1% lidocaine at the 4 and 8 o' clock positions around the cervix. Lidocaine (1 to 2 cc) should also be injected into the lip of the cervix where it is anticipated that the tenaculum or vulsellum forceps will be placed.
- NSAIDs can be given in advance of or immediately after the insertion in order to relieve cramping. However, studies do not indicate an analgesic result compared to placebo.

EQUIPMENT

- IUC (Mirena or ParaGard)
- Speculum
- Single-toothed tenaculum or atraumatic vulsellum forceps
- Betadine solution
- Uterine sound and cervical dilator
- Hemostatic agent for tenaculum site

TECHNIQUES

General Preparation

1. Premedication with ibuprofen (600 to 800 mg) may also help decrease the discomfort associated with insertion.

2. Prior to insertion of either IUC, it is necessary to perform a careful bimanual examination to confirm uterine position and exclude possible pelvic infection.
3. Results of recent previous screening for STIs should be available for patients considered at risk.
4. Insert the speculum and examine the cervix for signs of acute infection (mucopus).
5. Swab the cervix with Betadine.
6. Paracervical block as described above may be used at this time. If using a paracervical block, anesthetize the anterior or posterior lip of the cervix prior to tenaculum placement.
7. Grasp the lip of the cervix with the tenaculum. Asking the patient to cough while slowly closing the tenaculum will help make this step less painful.
8. Use gentle traction on the tenaculum to straighten the uterine axis.
9. Sound the uterus. Uterine length between 6 and 10 cm is required for IUC insertion.
10. Should you encounter resistance in sounding the uterus, do not use excessive force. Cervical dilators can be used to make passage of the sound easier.

Copper IUC (TCu380A, ParaGard) Insertion

1. Remove ParaGard from the packaging using sterile technique. Fold the horizontal arms of the device toward the stem and advance the insertion device over the arms using your other hand.
2. If the device is loaded within the sterile package, sterile gloves are not necessary. To do this, place the package on a clean, flat surface and open the bottom half of the package. Insert the white rod into the insertion sleeve until it meets the base of the intrauterine device (IUD). While holding the insertion sleeve with one hand put pressure up against the arms of the IUD until it arcs slightly. Use two fingers to bend the horizontal arms of the device toward the stem through the packaging. Withdraw the insertion sleeve slightly while continuing to bend the arms through the package. When the insertion sleeve has been withdrawn past the arms, gently advance the insertion device over the arms (twirling it slightly helps), thus loading the device (Figs. 21.2–21.5).
3. Advance the insertion sleeve only as far as necessary to ensure loading.
4. Adjust the blue flange on the insertion tubing so that the distance from the top of the loaded ParaGard to the flange is equal to the uterine depth.
5. Ensure that the T is in the same horizontal plane as the flange by rotating the insertion sleeve.
6. While applying gentle traction on the tenaculum pass ParaGard through the cervix up to the uterine fundus. At this point the blue flange should abut the cervical os.
7. Hold the solid white rod steady as you *withdraw* the insertion sleeve 1 cm (until it touches the ring hole of the insertion rod) to release the IUC high in the fundus. DO NOT push the solid white rod further into the uterus.
8. Gently advance the insertion sleeve toward the uterine fundus until mild resistance is noted to ensure placement of the IUC high in the fundus.
9. Slowly remove the solid white rod first, followed by the insertion sleeve.
10. Cut the IUC strings to approximately 3 cm.
11. Use ultrasound to ensure correct placement should there be any question as to fundal placement.

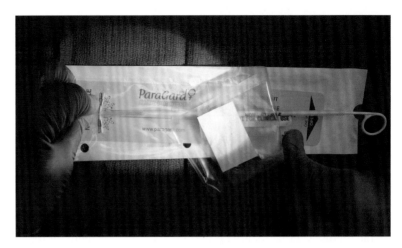

FIGURE 21.2 ● Preparing to load cross of the "T" into the sleeve of the inserter. Gentle pressure is placed at the underside of the "T" using the sleeve, causing the arm to bend downward.

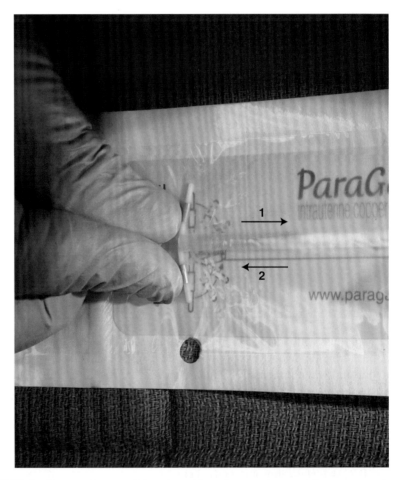

FIGURE 21.3 ● Forefinger and thumb positioned to put downward pressure on the arms, while immediately after this withdraw the sleeve (*1*) so that the arms can be tucked fully behind the shaft and the sleeve is brought forward again (*2*) to catch and tuck the arms.

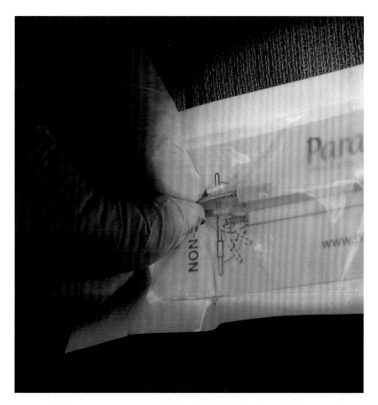

FIGURE 21.4 ● Copper T380 arms being tucked into inserter device.

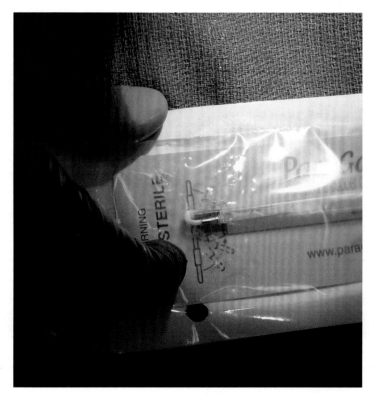

FIGURE 21.5 ● A loaded device.

Levonorgestrel-releasing IUC (LNg 20, Mirena) Insertion

1. Open package, then use sterile or clean examination gloves to complete loading process.
2. Release the strings tucked behind the slider on the Mirena insertion sleeve.
3. Push the slider away to the most proximal position on the insertion sleeve, closest to the Mirena.
4. Ensure the arms of the Mirena are in a horizontal plane with the insertion device.
5. Pull the strings of the Mirena down to load the complete IUC into the insertion sleeve. When fully loaded the entire IUC should be totally inside the insertion sleeve.
6. Pull the Mirena strings into the slit at the end of the insertion device.
7. Adjust the flange so that the distance from the top of the loaded Mirena to the flange equals the uterine depth.
8. While applying gentle traction on the tenaculum advance the insertion sleeve into the uterus until the flange is 1.5 cm from the cervical os.
9. Release the arms of the Mirena by pulling back on the slider to the horizontal mark on the insertion sleeve. Wait approximately 10 seconds to allow arms to deploy completely.
10. Gently advance the entire insertion sleeve until the flange abuts the cervical os (slight resistance should be felt at this point), ensuring placement of the Mirena in the fundus of the uterus (Fig. 21.6).
11. Hold the insertion sleeve securely as you pull the slider down toward you until a "click" is heard, releasing the Mirena strings.
12. Remove the insertion sleeve and cut the strings so that 2 to 3 cm protrude from the cervix (Fig. 21.7).

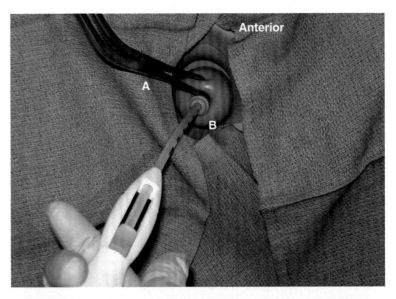

FIGURE 21.6 ● IUD insertion. **A:** Anterior cervix lip grasped with forceps after spraying area with local anesthetic. **B:** IUD insertion device (Mirena) being inserted to safety mark set by information gained from sounding.

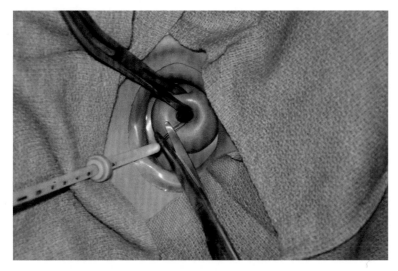

FIGURE 21.7 ● Cutting the strings (2.5 cm) at the end of procedure. It is best to cut the string when it is suspended in the sleeve as it is removed.

IUC Removal

1. Insert a speculum and visualize the strings extruding from the cervix.
2. Grasp the strings of the IUC with ring forceps and use gentle traction to remove the IUC.
3. If you are unable to remove the IUD with gentle traction, consider placement of a tenaculum so that the uterine axis may be straightened and facilitate removal of the IUC. Paracervical block may be used for more difficult removals.

Lost IUC

- Should the string not be visible, you can determine the location of the IUC with ultrasound.
- If the IUC is shown to be intrauterine, a cytobrush can be used to attempt to retrieve the strings and bring them back through the cervix.
- Alternatively, an alligator forceps can be gently inserted into the uterine cavity and the IUD retrieved with or without ultrasound guidance.
- Should the IUC have become imbedded in the wall of the uterus, hysteroscopy may be necessary to remove the IUC under direct visual guidance.
- Uterine perforation during insertion may result in intra-abdominal placement of the IUC. The IUC can be removed laparoscopically in this situation. Intra-abdominal placement of the ParaGard may ignite a severe inflammatory reaction with infection and abscess. Mirena, in contrast, is generally benign within the abdomen.

AFTERCARE

- Patient should return for an IUC string check following their next menses to ensure continued placement.
- Patient should be advised that they will experience cramping for a brief time following insertion.

- Again, patient should be aware of what to expect in the few months following insertion of either Mirena or ParaGard. These details should have been discussed prior to insertion as well.

CPT Codes
58300. Insertion of **IUD**
58301. Removal of **IUD**

PEARLS

- IUC is a very effective form of long-term birth control, but side effects can be inconvenient and lower the patient's confidence in the method. Preinsertion counseling can help prepare the patient for these side effects and enhance her confidence and perhaps her willingness to stick with the method despite the side effects.
- General preparation with adequate estimation of uterine length and proper insertion technique will minimize complications associated with IUC insertion.
- IUC removal is generally simple; however, it may require hysteroscopy or laparoscopy for removal under direct visual guidance in certain situations.

22

Office Urodynamics

Amy E. Wong and Eric R. Sokol

Evaluation of lower urinary tract disorders may be performed for patients presenting with:

- Storage symptoms: Frequency, nocturia, urgency, and urinary incontinence
- Voiding symptoms: Hesitancy, straining to void, poor stream, intermittent stream
- Postvoid symptoms: Incomplete emptying, postmicturition dribble

Initial evaluation includes a thorough medical history and review of medications that may affect the urinary tract. The patient can also keep a bladder diary and perform pad testing in order to provide further information about her urinary habits. Urinalysis should also be performed to exclude infection, hematuria, and metabolic abnormalities.

Before performing office urodynamics, several simple tests can be performed to assess etiology of urinary symptoms:

1. **Postvoid residual**
   - Can be assessed by either direct catheterization or ultrasonography.
   - Ultrasonography measurements have a standard error of 15% to 20%.
   - Perform within 10 minutes of a void.
   - Normal may be considered <50 mL and abnormal >200 mL. However, these values should be interpreted in the context of total voided volume and bladder capacity.

2. **Q-tip test**
   - Insert a sterile cotton-tipped stick lubricated with Xylocaine gel into the urethra up to, but not through the internal urethral sphincter (1 to 2 cm).
   - Have the patient cough or strain.
   - If the Q-tip moves >30 degrees, urethral hypermobility is suggested.

3. **Cough stress test**
   - Instruct the patient to cough vigorously with a full bladder.
   - Leakage at the time of cough tentatively supports the diagnosis of stress incontinence.
   - If leakage is not observed when supine, the test can be repeated in the upright position.
   - If the cough stress test is positive, the **Bonney test** can be performed by elevating the bladder neck by placing two fingers on either side of the urethra, pushing the bladder neck back into position. Have the patient cough; if no leakage occurs, the test is positive and suggestive of urethral hypermobility.

Advanced testing with urodynamics is recommended if the diagnosis is uncertain, the patient has failed prior therapy, or surgery is being considered. The purpose of urodynamic testing is to reproduce bladder filling, storage, and voiding symptoms while performing measurements to identify underlying causes for the symptoms.

Urodynamic testing includes:

1. **Simple uroflowmetry:** Measures urine flow rate and volume to identify abnormal voiding patterns in patients with suspected bladder outlet obstruction.
2. **Urethral pressure profile (UPP):** Evaluates ability of the urethra to prevent leakage.
3. **Cystometrogram (CMG):** Assesses for stress incontinence, detrusor activity, sensation, capacity, and compliance to evaluate the bladder's ability to store and release urine.
   a. *Single-channel* CMG detects abnormal bladder compliance and does not require special equipment, but does not provide absolute pressure measurements.
   b. *Multi-channel* CMG approximates the actual pressure exerted in the bladder by the activity of the detrusor muscle alone by subtracting the intra-abdominal pressure from the intravesical pressure.
      • Leak-point pressure is measured during multi-channel CMG and determines vesicular pressure when leakage occurs to assess for intrinsic sphincter deficiency.
4. **Pressure flow study:** Combines uroflow and CMG in same voiding event to show the relationship between bladder muscle strength and resulting flow to distinguish between bladder outlet obstruction and impaired detrusor function. It also evaluates for urethral relaxation before voiding.

RELEVANT ANATOMY

• Figure 22.1 (Anatomy of bladder)
• Urethra is approximately 4 cm in length and 6 mm in diameter
• Parasympathetic autonomic nervous system (S2–S4) performs detrusor contractions; sympathetic autonomic nervous system (T10–L2) performs storage during filling phase
• Figures 22.2 and 22.3 (muscular support of pelvic floor)

PATIENT POSITION

Dorsal lithotomy on the examination table or on the cystometric chair, unless otherwise indicated.

LANDMARKS

See relevant anatomy.

ANESTHESIA

None.

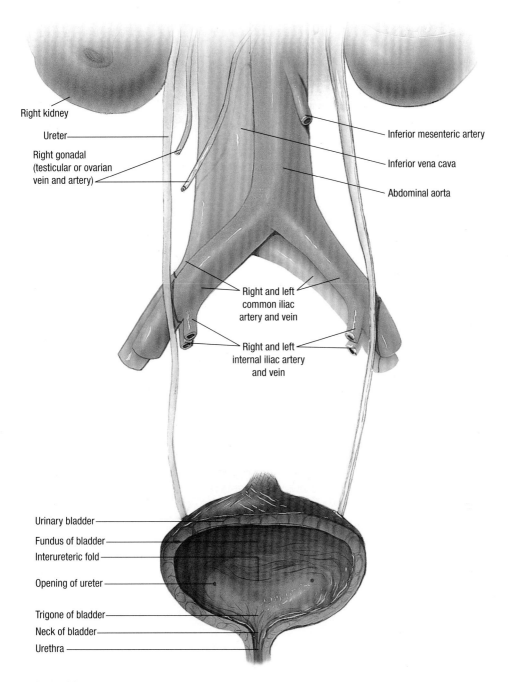

Right kidney

Ureter

Right gonadal
(testicular or ovarian
vein and artery)

Inferior mesenteric artery

Inferior vena cava

Abdominal aorta

Right and left
common iliac
artery and vein

Right and left
internal iliac artery
and vein

Urinary bladder

Fundus of bladder

Interureteric fold

Opening of ureter

Trigone of bladder

Neck of bladder

Urethra

FIGURE 22.1 ● Urinary bladder and collecting system. Asset provided by Anatomical Chart Co.

Superior view

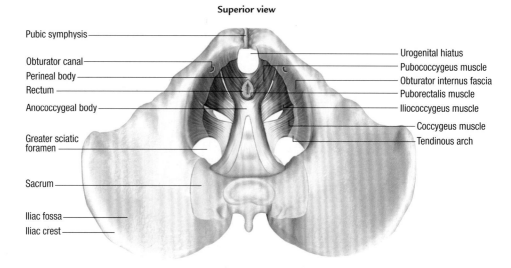

Pubic symphysis

Obturator canal
Perineal body
Rectum
Anococcygeal body

Greater sciatic
foramen

Sacrum

Iliac fossa
Iliac crest

Urogenital hiatus
Pubococcygeus muscle
Obturator internus fascia
Puborectalis muscle
Iliococcygeus muscle
Coccygeus muscle
Tendinous arch

FIGURE 22.2 ● Superior view of the pelvic wall and floor muscles. Asset provided by Anatomical Chart Co.

Inferior view

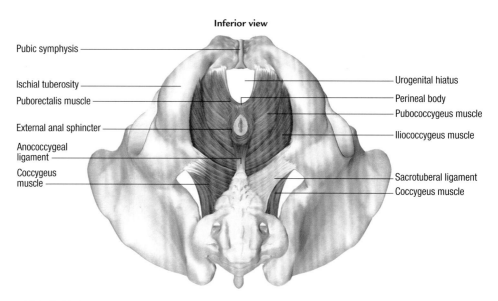

Pubic symphysis

Ischial tuberosity
Puborectalis muscle

External anal sphincter

Anococcygeal
ligament
Coccygeus
muscle

Urogenital hiatus

Perineal body
Pubococcygeus muscle

Iliococcygeus muscle

Sacrotuberal ligament
Coccygeus muscle

FIGURE 22.3 ● Inferior view of the pelvic wall and floor muscles. Asset provided by Anatomical Chart Co.

EQUIPMENT

- Sterile water or saline
- Betadine swabs
- Lubricant
- Straight catheter to empty bladder
- Uroflowmeter (for uroflow)
- Graduated large syringe (e.g., ≥60 mL) that is easy to pour fluid into (for simple cystometry)
- Pitcher to pour into the syringe (for simple cystometry)
- Stopwatch (for simple cystometry)
- Fluid-based, air-charged, or electronic catheters as available (for complex cystometry)
- Tape

TECHNIQUE

Simple Uroflowmetry ("Free Flow")

1. Patient to arrive with a full bladder.
2. Perform a cough stress test, both in the standing and squatting positions, if needed, for determining nature of incontinence.
3. Have patient empty bladder using a toilet or commode that directs the urine flow into a uroflowmeter.
4. Results reported: Peak flow rate (in mL/s), average flow, time to peak flow, voided volume, flow time, flow pattern.

Cystometrogram

- Single-channel (simple) cystometry (Fig. 22.4)
  1. Ask the patient to void and time with the stopwatch. Collect urine into a measuring hat to measure volume voided.
  2. Insert Foley or flexible catheter using sterile technique and measure postvoid urine volume.
  3. Attach graduated large syringe to the catheter.
  4. Pour sterile water at room temperature into the syringe and record times of:
     a. First desire to void
     b. Strong desire to void
     c. Sensation of urgency
     d. Sensation of reaching bladder capacity
     If strong urgency is noted, watch level of fluid in the graduated large syringe to see if it increases or fluctuates, which suggests detrusor overactivity.
  5. Remove catheter, and have patient cough and perform the Valsalva maneuver. Immediate loss of urine is suggestive of stress urinary incontinence (SUI).

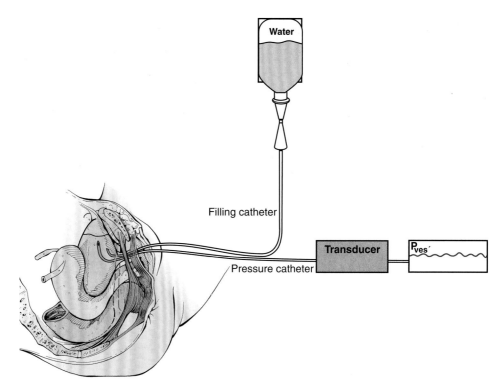

FIGURE 22.4 ● Typical setup for single-channel cystometry. Walters MD and Karram MM, eds. Urogynecology and reconstructive pelvic surgery. 2nd ed. St Louis: Mosby, 1999.

Urethral Pressure Profile

1. Have patient stand upright.
2. Fill bladder with a moderate amount of fluid (>50 mL).
3. Insert special urodynamic catheter that is used to simultaneously measure both urethral and bladder pressure (dual-tip catheter).
4. Slowly pull catheter through the urethra from the bladder (1 mm/s).
5. Assess the distance during which urethral pressure exceeds bladder pressure, which is the length of the continence zone or functional urethral length.
6. The urethral closure pressure (Pclo) can be calculated by subtracting the bladder pressure (Pves) from the urethral pressure (Pura). A maximum urethral closure pressure <20 cm of H_2O is diagnostic of intrinsic sphincter deficiency.
   - Multi-channel (complex) cystometrography
     1. Have patient empty bladder.
     2. Perform straight catheterization in sterile fashion to obtain postvoid residual.
     3. Insert pressure and filling catheter into bladder (may be two catheters or single–dual catheter) to measure intravesical pressure (Pves) and to fill bladder.
     4. Insert pressure catheter into upper vagina or rectum to approximate abdominal pressure (Pabd).
     5. Insert both catheters 6 to 10 cm and secure with tape.
     6. Infuse fluid (usually sterile water or saline) at a rate of around 50 mL/min. Record the volume infused and the pressure measurements continuously.

7. During filling, record times of:
   a. First sensation of filling
   b. First desire to void
   c. Strong desire to void
   d. Sensation of urgency
   e. Sensation of reaching bladder capacity
   f. Any leakage, if occurs
8. With a bladder volume of 200 or 300 mL, obtain the leak-point pressure. Ask the patient to cough with gradually increasing force (cough leak-point pressure) and finally to strain slowly (Valsalva) to increase intravesical pressure gradually. The lowest pressure at which leakage occurs is recorded as the Valsalva leak-point pressure. If the patient has moderate to severe prolapse, reduce the prolapse during this test.
9. If no detrusor overactivity is noted during filling, have the patient do provocative maneuvers at maximum capacity, such as coughing, to provoke uninhibited detrusor conditions.

Pressure Flow Study

1. Keep the bladder full at the completion of cystometrography. Or, if this test is to be performed separately from cystometrography, infuse bladder with normal saline until the patient feels she has reached her maximum bladder capacity.
2. Ask the patient to void and empty her bladder as completely as possible into a toilet or commode that directs the urine flow into a uroflowmeter while the urethral and rectal catheters are still in place.
3. Obtain flow rate from the uroflowmeter and detrusor pressure from the catheter measurement.
   a. Low flow rate and high detrusor pressure suggest bladder outlet obstruction. If the urethra does not concurrently relax, a neurologic problem is suggested, which can be evaluated with patch electromyography.
   b. Low flow rate and low detrusor pressure suggest an acontractile bladder. This should be further assessed with normal voiding dynamics (detrusor contraction, urethral relaxation, and urine flow).

AFTERCARE

- Normal activities may be resumed immediately after testing.
- Instruct the patient to drink plenty of fluids and void frequently.
- Caution the patient that she may have frequency, urgency, or a small amount of blood.
- The patient should call the physician if unable to void, pain, dysuria, or fever.
- Prophylactic antibiotics may be prescribed if desired by the physician.

CPT Codes

51736. Simple uroflowmetry (e.g., stop-watch flow rate, mechanical uroflowmeter)
51741. Complex uroflowmetry (e.g., calibrated electronic equipment)
51725. Simple CMG

51726.   Complex CMG
51772.   UPP studies or Valsalva leak-point pressures, any technique
57195.   Voiding pressure studies; bladder voiding pressure, any technique
57197.   Voiding pressure studies; intra-abdominal voiding pressure

PEARLS

- Normal values:
  - Postvoid residual: <50 mL
  - Flow rate: >15 mL/s in women older than 50 years and >25 mL/s in women younger than 50 years
  - First desire to void: 150 to 250 mL infused
  - Strong desire to void: >250 mL
  - Cystometric capacity: 400 to 600 mL
  - Valsalva leak-point pressure: Less than 60 cm H_2O diagnostic of intrinsic sphincter deficiency
  - Detrusor pressure during void: <50 cm H_2O
- Any uninhibited detrusor contractions during filling, even with provocation, are abnormal.
- All urodynamic studies require a negative dipstick, urine culture, or gram stain.
- Medications that may interfere with the test may be discontinued 1 to 2 days before testing at the discretion of the physician.
- Urodynamic testing is most frequently performed in a modified lithotomy position in the cystometric chair, but the standing position may be used as many patients with incontinence report this problem more when they are upright.
- Patients should be made as comfortable as possible to reproduce the normal voiding pattern.

23

Palpable Breast Mass

Amy E. Wong and Irene Wapnir

Background

The first step in the assessment of a palpable breast mass is a history and physical examination. Single masses especially with distinct borders are most often cysts of fibroadenomas. In a woman <30 to 35 years old without physical examination findings suggesting malignancy, such as a firm, immobile mass with irregular borders, it may be reasonable to have the patient return within 3 to 10 days after their next menstrual period to determine if the mass has regressed.

Alternatively, if a mass is suspected to be a simple cyst, aspiration may be performed in the office without prior radiologic evaluation. However, if the mass is suspected to be solid, diagnostic imaging should be performed. Ultrasound may be the first step in a woman <30 years old who has not had an aspiration. However, it is common today to consider a diagnostic mammogram, and/or MRI especially if there is a family history of breast cancer. Digital mammography exposes the patient to a lower radiation dose and is of superior quality, even for a woman with dense breasts, which may be more common in young women. In a woman >30 years old, diagnostic mammography, which includes the use of focused ultrasound to distinguish cystic from solid lesions, whether they are palpable or nonpalpable, is the study of choice.

Fine-needle aspiration (FNA) or core biopsy may also be performed by appropriately trained gynecologists or primary care physicians. If the lesion is a cyst, then aspiration should yield fluid with disappearance of mass. If lesion is solid, however, multiple passes with the needle should be performed to obtain cells for cytology. The advantage of FNA is the ease and quickness with which it can be performed. The largest concern with any needle biopsy is a false-negative result. Cytologic examinations often do not give definitive diagnoses such as fibroadenoma or phyllodes tumor, and also cannot distinguish between in situ and invasive cancer. Core-needle biopsy is more invasive, but can provide a more definitive histologic diagnosis. Regardless of the exact test performed, physical examination findings, imaging studies, and histologic results all need to be carefully integrated.

RELEVANT ANATOMY (Fig. 23.1)

- The breast is composed of 15 to 20 lobes, each composed of several lobules. Each lobe of the breast terminates in a major (lactiferous) duct (2 to 4 mm in diameter) which opens through a constructed orifice (0.4 to 0.7 mm in diameter) into the ampulla of the nipple.

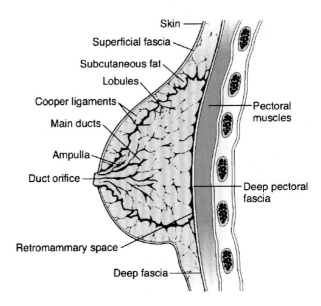

FIGURE 23.1 ● Breast anatomy. Breast anatomy in longitudinal section. From Daffner RH. *Clinical radiology: The essentials*, 3rd ed. Philadelphia, PA: Lippincott Williams & Wilkins, 2007.

- The suspensory ligaments of Cooper, fibrous bands of connective tissue, travel through the breast which insert perpendicularly into the dermis and provide structural support.
- The axillary tail of Spence extends laterally across the anterior axillary fold.
- The upper outer quadrant of the breast contains a greater volume of tissue than do the other quadrants.

PATIENT POSITION

- Supine on the examination table, arms usually at side.
- May place pillow under ipsilateral hemithorax.

LANDMARKS

- Palpate the location of the mass and identify the center.
- Isolate and stabilize the mass with fingers of the nondominant hand.
- Describe mass in relation to clock face and distance from areola.

ANESTHESIA

Local anesthesia with 1% lidocaine may be injected into the planned needle insertion site. While this is optional for cyst aspiration or FNA, it is necessary for a core biopsy. Alternatively, ethyl chloride can be sprayed on the skin over the planned needle insertion to numb it prior to biopsy.

Cyst Aspiration

EQUIPMENT

- Betadine swabs
- 25-gauge needle
- 10-mL syringe
- Sterile gauze pads
- Sterile adhesive bandage

TECHNIQUE

1. Cleanse site with Betadine.
2. Infiltrate skin with local anesthetic or spray planned aspiration site with ethyl chloride, if desired.
3. Attach needle to syringe.
4. Isolate and stabilize mass with fingers of nondominant hand.
5. Insert needle tip into cyst and aspirate fluid.
   a. If the fluid that is aspirated is not bloodstained, aspirate cyst to dryness and discard fluid as cytologic examination of fluid is not cost-effective.
   b. If the fluid is bloodstained, submit 2 mL of fluid for cytology.
   c. If the mass is solid, submit aspirated cells for cytologic analysis.
6. After aspiration, carefully palpate breast to exclude a residual mass. If one exists, perform ultrasound to exclude a persistent cyst, which should be reaspirated if present.

   For use in identifying breast cysts, probe frequency should be 10 MHz or higher. If this is not available in the office, the patient should be sent to facility where this is possible. (Note: The provider can only bill for image guidance if certi-fied to read *breast* ultrasounds.)
7. Apply a sterile adhesive bandage over the aspiration site.

CPT Code
19000.   Puncture aspiration of cyst of breast

Fine-needle Aspiration (FNA)

EQUIPMENT

- Betadine swabs
- 25-gauge needle
- 10-mL syringe
- 1% lidocaine (or other local anesthetic), optional
- Microscope slides (2) or CytoLyt
- 95% Ethanol fixative
- Sterile gauze pads
- Sterile adhesive bandage

TECHNIQUE (Fig. 23.2)

1. Cleanse skin with Betadine.
2. Infiltrate skin with local anesthetic, if desired.
3. Attach needle to syringe.
4. Isolate and stabilize mass with fingers of nondominant hand.
5. Insert needle tip into mass and apply suction while the needle is moved back and forth within the mass.
6. Once cellular material is seen at the hub of the needle, release suction and withdraw needle.
7. Express cellular material onto microscope slide and prepare both air-dried and 95% ethanol-fixed microscopy preparations for analysis.
8. Apply a sterile adhesive bandage over the aspiration site.

CPT Code

10021.   FNA without imaging guidance

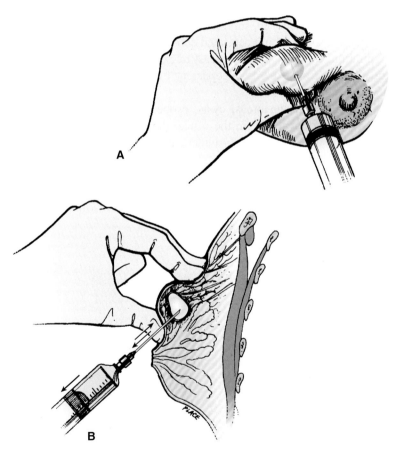

FIGURE 23.2 ● Needle aspiration of cystic breast mass. **A:** Needle is passed into cyst, which is stabilized as shown. **B:** The cyst contents are removed by gentle suction. LifeART image copyright © 2012 Lippincott Williams & Wilkins. All rights reserved.

Core-needle Biopsy

EQUIPMENT

- Ultrasound machine with probe frequency of 10 MHz or greater, optional
- Betadine swabs
- 14-gauge biopsy needle (e.g., Tru-Cut needle)
- Scalpel
- 1% lidocaine (or other local anesthetic)
- Specimen container containing formalin
- Sterile gauze pads
- Sterile adhesive bandage

TECHNIQUE (Fig. 23.3)

1. Cleanse skin with Betadine.
2. Infiltrate skin over the planned incision site with local anesthetic.
3. Isolate and stabilize mass with fingers of nondominant hand.
4. Make a 2- to 3-mm skin incision with the scalpel.
5. Place needle in mass repetitively to obtain three to six tissue specimens.
6. Compress breast for several minutes until hemostasis is achieved.
7. Apply a sterile adhesive bandage over the biopsy site.

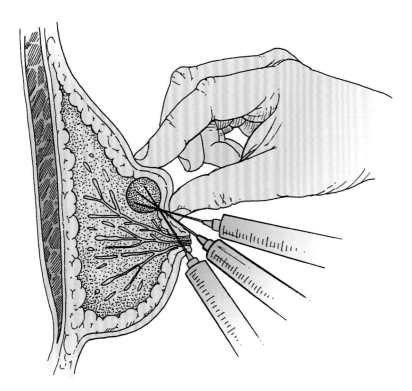

FIGURE 23.3 ● Fine-needle aspiration. The nondominant hand of the operator stabilizes the breast mass while multiple passes are made with the needle and syringe held in the dominant hand. LifeART image copyright © 2012 Lippincott Williams & Wilkins. All rights reserved.

AFTERCARE

- Pain is minimal and can be managed with an over-the-counter analgesic.
- Core biopsy can cause bruising on the breast during the first week after biopsy.
- Complications are rare, but excessive swelling, redness, bleeding, or other drainage may indicate an infection or bleeding within the mass/biopsy site.

CPT Code

19100. Biopsy of breast; percutaneous, needle core, not using imaging guidance

PEARLS

- The two cardinal rules of safe cyst aspiration are: (1) The mass must disappear completely after aspiration, and (2) the fluid must not be bloodstained. If either of these conditions is not met, then ultrasound, needle biopsy, and perhaps excisional biopsy are recommended.
- After FNA or core biopsy, the patient should be examined in 4 to 6 weeks to ensure that the cyst has not reappeared.
- Referral to a surgical specialist should be performed for any persistent or recurrent breast mass.

Further Readings

American Society for Colposcopy and Cervical Pathology, Mayeaux EJ, Cox JT, eds. *Modern Colposcopy Textbook and Atlas,* 3rd ed. Philadelphia: Lippincott Williams & Wilkins, 2011.

Baird TL, Castleman LD, Hyman AG, et al. *Clinician's Guide for Second-Trimester Abortion*, 2nd ed. Chapel Hill: Ipas, 2007. (www.ipas.org)

Baggish MS, Valle RF, Guedj H, eds. *Hysteroscopy: Visual Perspectives of Uterine Anatomy, Physiology, and Pathology*, 3rd ed. Philadelphia: Lippincott Williams & Wilkins, 2007.

Bent AE, Cundiff GW, Swift SE, eds. *Ostergard's Urogynecology and Pelvic Floor Dysfunction*, 6th ed. Philadelphia: Lippincott Williams & Wilkins, 2007.

Berek JS, ed. *Berek and Novak's Gynecology*, 15th ed. Philadelphia : Lippincott Williams & Wilkins, 2011.

Curtis MG, Overholt S, Hopkins MP, eds. *Glass' Office Gynecology*, 6th ed. Philadelphia: Lippincott Williams & Wilkins, 2005.

Emans SJ, Laufer MR, eds. *Emans, Laufer, Goldstein's Pediatric and Adolescent Gynecology*, 6th ed. Philadelphia: Lippincott Williams & Wilkins, 2011.

Mayeaux EJ, ed. *Essential Guide to Primary Care Procedures*, 1st ed. Philadelphia: Lippincott Williams & Wilkins, 2009.

Paul M, Lichtenberg S, Borgatta L, et al., eds. *Management of Unintended and Abnormal Pregnancy: Comprehensive Abortion Care*, 1st ed. Philadelphia: Wiley-Blackwell, 2009.

Index

Note: Page numbers followed "*f*" denote figures; those followed by "*t*" denote tables.